TROPICAL HYGIENE FOR SCHOOLS

TROPICAL HYGIENE
FOR SCHOOLS

BY

E. J. EVANS, B.Sc. (LOND.), L.C.P.

Revised, with additions,

BY

CLEMENT C. CHESTERMAN, O.B.E., M.D., F.R.C.P., D.T.M.&H.

Author of *Tropical Dispensary Handbook*
Lecturer on Tropical Hygiene, University of London
Institute of Education

LUTTERWORTH PRESS
LONDON

New edition 1966
Second impression 1966
Third impression 1966
Fourth impression 1967
Fifth impression 1968
Copyright © 1966 Lutterworth Press

7188 0946 7

Printed in Great Britain by Page Bros. (Norwich) Ltd.

REVISER'S PREFACE

I am glad to continue the task of providing a school text-book which covers the curriculum for the General Certificate in Health Science. As in former editions it aims at including the hygiene which the educated man and woman in the tropics need to know. They need it to help them co-operate with the sanitary authorities; they need it to bring up a family; they need it if they are to become useful leaders or members of their community.

To include what is necessary for the tropics this book has to be very different from a hygiene manual for non-tropical countries. In these, health can be maintained almost without a knowledge of disease. Ventilation, exercise and right feeding prevent many of the diseases common there. In the tropics, germs and parasites abound; they may attack anyone— even if he takes all those general precautions. He needs, as well as ordinary health teaching, such information as, for instance, how a hook-worm enters the body; how malaria is carried; and what diseases the village pig may give him.

Mr. E. J. Evans laid an excellent foundation for teaching all aspects of hygiene, and it is hoped that this edition is an up-to-date fulfilment of his aims. In this task I wish to acknowledge the help and guidance received from my colleague Professor L. J. Lewis, Head of the Department of Education in Tropical Areas, of the London University Institute of Education.

CONTENTS

vii

LIST OF ILLUSTRATIONS

GENERAL HYGIENE

Chapter 1

INTRODUCTION

The subject of Hygiene and Sanitation is a very important one in all countries, but is especially so in tropical ones where the warmth and dampness, together with ignorance of the laws of health, make it easy for disease to spread.

Hygiene is the science which teaches us how to keep healthy. Hygiene teaches us the laws of health, especially as these are applied to individual people.

Sanitation is the art by which the laws of health are applied to a number of people living in the same place, that is, to the community. It deals with Public Health, which is usually a Government undertaking.

Health and Disease.—We say a person is healthy when all the parts of his body are doing their work properly. For this it is of course necessary that the various parts should be properly made to start with. When a man's organs are defective, or when for some cause or other they are not working properly, we say he has some disease.

Physiology.—The subject of Hygiene does not actually include the study of the body and its various parts. But as the aim of Hygiene is to keep the body healthy it is necessary to have some knowledge of how the body works and what it requires to keep it going. We need therefore to know a little about the form and structure of our bodies (Anatomy), and about the way the various parts function (Physiology).

THE BODY

Living Things, whether they be plants or animals, may vary very much in size and shape and mode of life, but they are all alike in many ways.

They all need much the same sorts of food in order to grow and multiply and to give them energy for work. They all absorb some of the food and have waste products which they must get rid of by excretion. They must be able to reproduce themselves by dividing or budding off, or by spores, seeds, eggs or young. They must be able to respond to changes of temperature or moisture in their surroundings (environment). They should be able to recover from minor injuries and disease.

To do all this the living thing or organism must have many different parts or organs, each with a special job or function to perform. Many organs may work together at one task, making what we call a System. In a healthy body all the systems work in harmony together for the benefit of the whole. One eye does not want to look to the right while the other looks to the left. One leg does not try to go forward while the other goes backward.

SYSTEMS OF THE BODY

Cutaneous System. The skin encloses and protects all the organs of the body. It lets heat in when we want to warm ourselves and cools us by sweating when we are too hot.

It contains the delicate nerve endings by which we know the touch or feel of things and their size and shape, also feelings of pain and pressure, heat and cold.

The Skeletal System. The bones or Skeleton give

shape and strength to the body and limbs. They are linked together by joints which are like hinges and permit movement.

The Muscular System makes up the meat on our bones. When the muscles pull they bend or straighten our joints and so move eyes, tongue, face and limbs, etc. They can act only when they get a message through the nerves.

The Nervous System, with the brain, the spinal cord and the nerves directs and controls all our bodily movement and sensation. Messages go up to the brain through the sensory nerves giving it news of our feeling or position and orders go out from the brain by the motor nerves to muscles and organs. There is also an automatic nervous system, not controlled by the conscious brain which regulates the various functions of the body which go on by themselves without our knowing it, such as the beat of the heart, etc.

The Circulatory System. The heart pumps the blood from its right half through the lungs and back to its left half. This is called the Lesser Circulation and serves to purify the blood in the lungs before it is pumped round the body in the Greater Circulation. This, sometimes called the Systemic Circulation, starts in the great throbbing arteries from the left half of the heart, through the smaller and smaller arteries to the minute hair-like tubes or capillaries among the body cells and back via the bluish veins to the right half of the heart again.

The Respiratory System. The air we breathe passes down the windpipe and bronchial tubes to the lungs. Here it comes into close contact with the blood which has come back by the veins from the whole body bringing the carbon dioxide with it. The air gives up oxygen to this blood and takes the CO_2 away from it.

The Digestive System. The mouth, the throat, the

gullet, the stomach and the large and small bowel form a long tube. In it the food we take is mixed with various juices, digested and partly absorbed and passed on to the liver for further preparation or storage. The indigestible portion passes out in the stools (fæces). Defæcation, Urination, Expiration and Perspiration form our Excretory System.

The Urinary System provides for a sort of filtering of the blood by the kidneys. These two organs allow the urine to pass down through the ureters to the bladder to await periodical discharge through the urethra.

The Endocrine System comprises a number of glands (e.g. the thyroid, the pituitary and the adrenals) which secrete juices into the blood. These regulate many body functions.

The Reproductive System provides for mating and the growth of the child in the mother's womb. There the minute egg from one of her two ovaries, fertilized by the sperm from the father's testis, grows into a baby in ten lunar months. Its food comes from the mother's blood through the umbilical cord, but after birth from her milk.

ILLNESS

When all these organs and systems do not work well for some reason or other, we feel ill and may have aches and pains or fever. We may be able to " sleep it off " and feel better next day for the body is often able to put itself right again without any medicine. When it cannot do this we may get seriously ill and our friends may get worried. People who have not learned about health and hygiene will say that perhaps we have forgotten to wear a charm, or have broken a tabu or that someone has cursed us or cast a spell or the evil eye on us. Others may say that the spirit of an ancestor is angry with us. Or they may go to the witch doctor to ask him to find

out who has bewitched us. So they may start asking
Who? has caused it instead of What? and they often
get the wrong answer.

If a motor car does not work properly we don't ask
Who? has put a juju on it. We ask a good mechanic
to examine it and find out *What?* is wrong with it. We
shall find that similar reasons cause bad working in cars
and bodies.

In a MOTOR CAR	BAD WORKING *may be due to:*	*In our* BODIES
From factory or garage	1. Defective parts	From parents or at birth
Wear and tear	2. Worn parts	Ageing and disease
Accident and strain	3. Damaged parts	Injuries and strain
Wrong kind or lack	4. Fuel or Food	Wrong kind or lack
Dirt and rust	5. Things picked up	Germs and worms

PREVENTION OF ILLNESS

How can we prevent these five kinds of illness?

1. **Hereditary Disease** may come from our parents,
e.g. Sickling is due to defective blood. **Congenital
Disease** may be present at birth owing to harm to the
child while in the womb, e.g. hole in the heart or club
foot. We can't do much to prevent.

2. **Ageing** and wearing out through disease causes
bad working of both body and mind and our best hope
is to put off or escape these through healthy living.

3. **Accidents** and injuries we can hope to avoid. We
can learn a little about First Aid when they do happen.

4. **Nutritional Diseases** can be avoided by knowing
what foods are best and the right amount and variety
in our diet.

5. **Infectious or Communicable Diseases** due to germs
and worms are caught direct from person to person, or
through insect bites and lack of hygiene. We can learn
to avoid these by clean air, clean food, clean water, clean
bodies, clean clothes, clean houses and clean villages,
good sanitation of towns and protection from insects.
We can also use preventive inoculations and medicines.

B

Chapter 2

AIR

Air is the most important thing the body requires. A man can live some days without water, and some weeks without food, but cannot live five minutes without air. It is the first necessity of life.

Composition.—Air is a gas which is a mixture of other gases. These are Oxygen, Nitrogen and Carbon Dioxide.

The proportions in which the chief gases are present in pure air may be taken as:

Nitrogen 79 parts in every 100 parts.

Oxygen 21 parts in every 100 parts.

Carbon Dioxide, a trace.

Air also contains variable quantities of Water (in the form of vapour), Ammonia and, in certain districts, suspended matter.

Nitrogen.—This forms the bulk of the air, practically four parts out of five. It is a gas without colour, taste, or smell. It is of no use to the body and will not keep animals alive or even flames burning. A person who breathed pure nitrogen would die of suffocation, that is, of lack of oxygen; he would not be poisoned.

Oxygen.—This forms one part in five of the air, and is the most important part of it for human and animal life. It has no colour, taste, or smell. It is the one gas necessary for all breathing and burning. If the air had more oxygen in it things would burn much more brightly and quickly, but nature has provided that the air should be diluted by nitrogen.

Carbon Dioxide.—This is a colourless gas with a faint smell and taste. It is a heavy gas and will sink to the bottom of a bottle containing it. It is therefore found in greater quantities near the ground than higher up in the air. It is often written CO_2 for short.

Carbon dioxide is produced in great quantities by three causes, Burning, Breathing and Decay. It is continually being put into the air. How is it then that the air does not gradually become full of carbon dioxide? Millions of people and animals are breathing it out and millions of fires and lamps are producing it. The explanation is that trees and all green plants make use of it. The gas (CO_2) contains carbon and oxygen united together. It enters the minute pores of the green leaves where it is absorbed by the green colouring matter (chlorophyll) which they contain. When sunlight or any bright artificial light falls on the leaf, the energy in the light breaks the bond between the carbon and the oxygen of the CO_2. The carbon then combines with the water in the sap to make sugar or starch to feed the plant, but the oxygen escapes into the air again. Thus living plants purify the air.

We may look upon the above gases, Nitrogen, Oxygen and Carbon Dioxide, as the ordinary parts of pure air. We have now to learn something about the other gases which are found in the air.

Water Vapour.—Water is always present in the air in the form of an invisible gas. The hotter it is the more water the air will hold.

To prove this obtain a glass of cold water. Soon you will notice a film of moisture form on the outside of the glass. This has come from the air. The air near the glass gets cold and cannot hold the water it held before. It therefore has to drop some. The air in the tropics is often very full of water and the above experiment is very easy to perform. If a glass of iced water is placed on a table-cloth the moisture in the air settles so quickly on the outside of the glass that it runs down and wets the cloth.

Our comfort depends greatly upon the amount of moisture in the air. This is called the " humidity " of the air. Very humid air is uncomfortable.

Impurities.—The following impurities are sometimes found in air.

Ammonia.—This is a gas which, when well diluted with air, has a rather pleasant smell. When dissolved in water it forms the Ammonia we can buy in the stores. It is a poison, but is never present in the air in sufficient quantities to harm anyone. But it does indicate a danger because it is produced by decaying animal and vegetable matter.

Suspended Matter.—If a ray of sunlight is allowed to pass through a narrow opening into a dark room the air will be seen to be full of " motes ". Some are too small to be seen. They may be either *organic*, that is from animals or plants or matter formed by them, or *inorganic* (mineral), and they may be dangerous to health.

Organic matter may be minute specks of the skin, hair or feathers of man, animals or birds, or germs from their breath or excreta. Also the pollen of grasses and flowers and the dust of hay, cotton or other fibres.

Inorganic matter consists of particles of sand, lime, dust, soot or smoke. In mines, coal dust and rock dust often cause lung trouble.

Impure Gases.—These may come from factory chimneys in industrial areas and consist mainly of sulphurous fumes. They are also given off from swamps and mud banks in creeks and mangrove areas. In countries where coal gas is used for burning in houses the gas is sometimes found in the air because of leaking pipes. Coal gas contains a very poisonous gas called Carbon Monoxide (CO).

The Effect on Air of Breathing.—We have been told that ordinary pure air has the following composition:

Oxygen . . . . 21 per cent
Nitrogen . . . . 79 ,, ,,
Carbon Dioxide . . trace
Moisture . . . . variable

Breathed out or expired air is composed as follows:

Oxygen . . . . 17 per cent
Nitrogen . . . . 79 ,, ,,
Carbon Dioxide . . 4 ,, ,,
Moisture . . . . saturated
Organic matter . . traces

Noticing these figures we come to this conclusion:

1. The Nitrogen remains the same.
2. The Oxygen decreases.
3. The Carbon Dioxide increases.

In addition:

4. The temperature of the air is raised.
5. The expired air is full of moisture (saturated).
6. It contains now organic impurities thrown off by the lungs.

Let us notice one or two things:

(*a*) The oxygen gets less while the carbon dioxide increases. The explanation is as follows: In the body cells a sort of slow burning takes place. The oxygen of the air is carried to the cells by the blood. It unites with the carbon in our food and forms carbon dioxide. This is sometimes expressed as: $C + O_2 = CO_2$. The blood brings this CO_2 to the lungs to get rid of it.

(*b*) The temperature of the air is raised. Our bodies usually have a temperature between 98° and 99°, and expired air is raised to about 96°.

(*c*) The organic matter escaping from the lungs is another impurity produced by breathing. It may contain germs of disease.

(d) When you breathe on a piece of glass, moisture settles on it. The glass has been standing in ordinary air as the tumbler of iced water did; yet no water formed on it from the air until you breathed on it. This shows that there is more moisture in breathed-out air. There is as much moisture in it as it can hold; such air is then said to be " saturated ". The moisture breathed out is the chief cause of stuffiness in a crowded room.

From the above we see that there is need to change the air of a room in order to keep it fit for us to breathe. Every breath spoils the air to some extent. A person who breathes air which has already been breathed does not get his fair share of life-giving oxygen, but gets more than his share of CO_2 and organic matter and these do him harm.

It has been found that a man may breathe one part of CO_2 in 100 parts of air without any bad effects, though more than this would give headache and make him drowsy. So we see that the gas is not very poisonous.

When, however, we examine air which has been

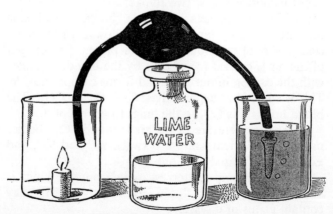

Fig. 1.—CO_2 turns Lime Water milky.

breathed, we find that a man cannot breathe it without discomfort even when it is mixed with a good deal of fresh air. This is due to the fact that breathed air is warm and moist, and contains CO_2 and organic impurities which, even if they come from healthy people, are bad to breathe into the lungs.

Fainting, sickness, and headache produced by crowds are due not only to heat, moisture, and carbon dioxide, but also to fatigue and exhaustion.

The arranging of doors, windows and chimneys, so as to supply good air and remove bad, is called *Ventilation*.

The amount of air which has to flow into a room ten feet high with a ten foot by ten foot floor with one person in it should be enough to fill the room again every twenty minutes. If there are four people in the room, they need a whole roomful of air every five minutes in a room of this size.

SOME EXPERIMENTS ON AIR

1. To test for Carbon Dioxide.—Place some clear lime water in a glass. With an enema syringe, pump air through this as follows:

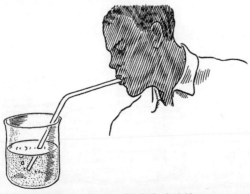

Fig. 2.—To show CO_2 in Expired Air.

First pump ordinary air through it. As this contains only a trace of CO_2 the lime water will not become cloudy unless the pumping is continued for a very long time.

Now burn a candle in another glass or mug, and pump the air from this vessel through the lime water. The lime water then turns milky. The milkiness is due to chalk which the CO_2 makes with the lime.

2. To show we breathe out Carbon Dioxide.—Blow into some clear lime water through a straw or other tube. The water turns milky.

3. To show the proportion of Oxygen in Air.—

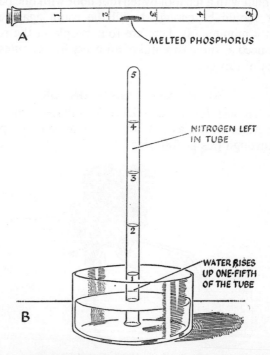

Fig. 3.—(A) Phosphorus absorbing Oxygen.   (B) Water taking its place

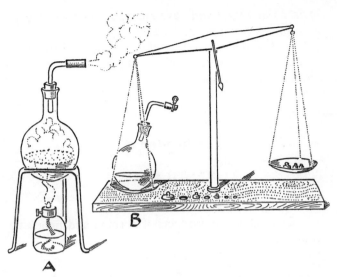

Fig. 4.—(A) Expelling the Air by boiling.   (B) Weighing the Flask.

Obtain a glass tube about an inch wide and 2 or 3 feet long, corked at one end and closed at the other. Drop a piece of phosphorus into the tube and cork up. Gently warm the phosphorus which melts and absorbs the oxygen in the tube. Now place the tube upright in water and take out the cork under water. It will be found that the water will rise one-fifth of the tube to take the place of the oxygen. The gas left is nitrogen.

4. To prove Air has Weight.—Take a glass round-bottomed flask containing a little water. Fit in a cork with a short glass tube inserted through it. Fix on a piece of rubber tubing, as shown in sketch. Have a rubber tubing clip ready. Boil the water to drive out the air. Then clip the tube. Now weigh the flask. This gives the weight of the flask and water. When cool, open the clip. Air rushes in and fills the flask. Weigh again. The weight will have increased owing to the air admitted, proving air has weight.

We know that air has weight when we feel the force of the wind. It is the weight of the air which makes it possible for birds and aeroplanes to fly in it.

Chapter 3

VENTILATION

The Objects of Ventilation are:

1. To remove the products of burning and breathing from the room.

2. To replace them with pure air.

PURIFICATION OF AIR

The air is rendered pure by:

1. The action of plants and trees (see page 7).

2. The falling of rain. This washes away dust (suspended impurities), both organic and inorganic, and makes the air fresh.

3. The oxygen in the air, which changes the organic impurities in the air and renders them harmless.

4. The sun. Nearly all germs exposed to its direct rays are soon killed.

Hot Air Rises.—Another natural property of gases made use of in ventilation is the fact that hot air rises. When gas is heated it expands and becomes lighter than the colder gas around. The air near fires, and air that has been breathed out, is foul or dirty air. It is lighter than pure air because it is warm. The dirty air in a room rises and finds its way out through any hole in the wall or in the ceiling. Cool pure air from outside takes its place. The fact that warm air rises also causes winds (see page 196).

METHODS OF VENTILATION

Ventilation may be *artificial* or *natural*. Artificial ventilation which is used for cinemas and other halls depends on fans and pumps which force the air to circulate by mechanical means.

1. The pure air may be forced into the room, usually by electric fans.

2. The bad air may be sucked out of the room. Here again fans are used and the impure air is driven through tubes near the roof.

3. As commonly used, electric fans and punkahs can hardly be called methods of ventilation. They set the air of the room in motion and in tropical houses produce a refreshing current of air, but they do not of themselves drive out the bad air and supply pure.

4. Air-conditioning is the name given to the perfected system of ventilation by which air is warmed or cooled, moistened or dried, to produce conditions regarded as ideal for human comfort and health. In the tropics, air-conditioned rooms tend to be a little chilly; they should not be made quite as cool and dry as would be ideal in other parts of the world.

Natural Means of Ventilation.—In the tropics we make use of the natural properties of air, aided by simple apparatus.

The ventilation of houses in Europe is, in one sense, more difficult than in the tropics, where the temperature of the air is much the same inside the house as outside and so we may admit a breeze without troubling about draughts. In Europe the temperature outside might be, say, 32°, and the inside temperature 65° or 70°. Fresh air must be allowed in, and all the fresh air available is cold; if a current of it blew steadily on to anyone, he would possibly get a chill. Therefore special means have to be used to see that the incoming air is either warmed or directed away from people inside.

Most tropical houses are so built that sufficient ventilation can be obtained by means of the doors and

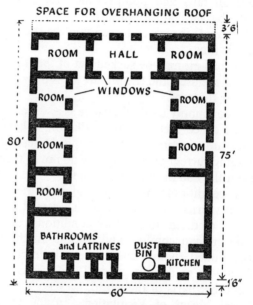

SPACE FOR OVERHANGING ROOF

3'6"

ROOM   HALL   ROOM

— WINDOWS —

ROOM   ROOM

80'   ROOM   ROOM   75'

ROOM

BATHROOMS and LATRINES   DUST BIN   KITCHEN   1'6"

60'

Fig. 5.—A Properly Planned Compound.

windows. Most of the houses have an opening between the top of the walls and the eaves of the roof. This space provides an outlet for bad air; the inlets are the doors and windows. This simple method of opening doors and windows and allowing the breeze to flow through is very effective.

The winds can purify the air in the house only if the building is properly arranged. The rooms themselves

must have a certain amount of window area. This is
regulated by law; the windows must be one-tenth the
area of the floor. This is a minimum figure and better
houses have twice as much window space. The windows
should be at opposite sides of the room to allow the
breeze to pass through the room. When the house
consists of several rooms, they must be placed so that
as many of them as possible have the wind blowing
through them (see Fig. 5).

Objections are sometimes made to this use of
windows:

(1) At night the house would not be safe from thieves
were windows and doors open. That is true, but health
is so important that some plan must be found. Let the
door be locked at night, and the windows made, not
of plain wood or glass, but of strong wire. Expanded
metal or arc mesh is now largely used and will protect
from thieves and yet allow air to pass through. Jalousies
are better than plain wood. Many houses have two sets
of shutters to the windows; one made of wire or
glass, opening inwards, and the other made of wooden
louvre or jalousy, opening outwards.

(2) But it may be asked, What about tornadoes or
hurricanes? The windows must be shut. But the violent
rain only lasts a short time, and the windows should be
opened when it is over. Moreover in ordinary storms
the rain often comes from one side of the house only,
and the other side is not affected.

The compound in which each house is built must
also be properly planned. If everybody buys a small
piece of land and builds a house to cover it, the wind
will have no chance to ventilate the houses. In some
areas laws have been made that only a certain part of
the land bought may be covered with buildings. This
gives a good chance to put the latrine, the kitchen and

the dust bin some distance from the house. Around such a compound a fence which allows wind to pass is, of course, better than a wall.

Town planning is so arranged that the wind can circulate among the houses. Regulating building in

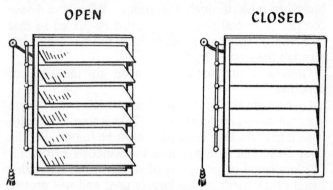

Fig. 6.—A modern glass louvre.

this way has improved many tropical towns, and nowadays the chiefs of towns which do not come under the regulations sometimes ask to have their towns planned for them.

The planting of bushes and trees is clearly a very useful way of purifying the air; but they must be so arranged that the wind has free access to the houses. Trees that are well grown, for instance, should have their lower branches cut away.

Ventilation of Modern Houses.—Tropical towns now have some houses built on the European plan; certain internal rooms may have need of special ventilation. There are also churches, halls and schools which, when crowded with people and artificially lighted at night, need ventilating apparatus. We give here a few of the methods used in the ventilation of modern houses.

(*a*) One or more of the panes may be changed for louvre slips which may be opened or closed by a lever These are best made with glass.

(*b*) A *hinged pane* may be inserted. This will direct air from outside up into the room.

(*c*) Many small tropical houses with board windows and doors can be greatly improved by the extremely simple step of cutting off a few inches of the door and window, top and bottom. Nobody can claim that this will help thieves to enter, but bad air can get out and the breeze can get in through such openings.

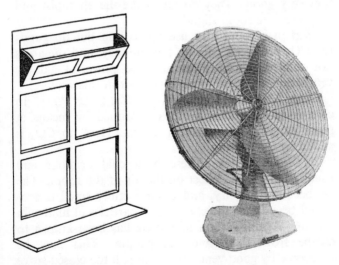

Fig. 7.—Ventilation by a Hinged Pane.

Fig. 8.—Electric Fan

(*d*) *Modern methods of ventilation.* Electric fans can be used to keep the air moving and thus make one feel cooler. If they are fixed into a window high near the ceiling they can suck the hot air out and draw in cooler air from the ground level.

(*e*) *Air conditioning* is done by machines which pump cooled and dried air into the room.

The Effect of Lights and Heating.—Kerosene lamps, candles and coal gas use up oxygen in burning and produce CO_2 and water vapour. It has been calculated that a candle burning uses up half as much air as a man. A kerosene lamp equals a man, and gas-lamps equal more than two men. If, therefore, we have lamps burning in our rooms more fresh air will have to be supplied.

Electric Lamps do not use up oxygen and are therefore very good. They do not make the air moist and only heat the room slightly.

Fires in a room also use up oxygen but do good; the CO_2 produced goes up the chimney, and the air is not spoiled much. Fires also are powerful aids to ventilation and tend to purify the air in this way.

Other Methods of Heating.—1. *Hot-water Pipes.* In cold countries rooms are often warmed by means of pipes carrying hot water or steam. Here no CO_2 is added by the heating.

2. *Closed Stoves.* These burn coal or coke and usually have a bad effect on the air of the room. The air becomes too dry, and often a stuffy smell is produced because of the charring of particles of matter in the air. Again, carbon monoxide has been known to escape from them and kill people. This may be overcome by good ventilation, but still the closed stove tends to spoil the air.

Overcrowding.—We are now able to understand one danger of having our rooms full of people. In tropical countries the rooms have so many doors and windows that there is little chance of having insufficient air during the day. Besides, the heat gives us a warning; we would not allow ourselves the discomfort of overcrowding. At night, however, there is a danger. The custom is to close tightly all doors and windows for fear of thieves. Many people sleep in the same room, and as they are unconscious and do not notice the badness of the air they think nothing is wrong.

The effects of overcrowding, however, are very serious. If the air cannot be changed sufficiently to allow every person sufficient fresh air, it follows that they must breathe the same air over and over again. What are the consequences?

1. They get insufficient oxygen. The blood therefore is not well purified. The " soldiers " of the bodily town are badly fed and get weak; disease becomes more likely. This may not take place in one night, or even in a month or year, but the effect will surely be seen in time. People who live and sleep in overcrowded rooms are generally feeble.

2. They run a great risk of catching infectious diseases from each other, especially those which are air-borne like sore throats, measles, mumps and influenza. Tuberculosis, meningitis and pneumonia are often caught through overcrowding.

Chapter 4

WATER

About three-quarters of the body is made of water, so it is, next to oxygen, the most important of our needs. A sufficient amount of water is especially necessary for removing refuse from the body in perspiration, urine and fæces.

Water is taken into the body, not only by drinking,

but also as a part of our solid food. Meat and fish contain about 75 per cent of water: green vegetables about 90 per cent.

A supply of pure water is very important as it is by water that many disease germs and poisons find entrance into the body. What do we mean by "pure" water? For our purposes, water is *pure* so long as it has no injurious effects upon our bodies. Such water may contain a good many things dissolved in it. We ought to call it "good" water rather than "pure".

"Good" Water should have the following properties:
1. It should be clear, colourless and sparkling.
2. It should have no smell or taste.
3. It should be free from germs of disease.

The Uses of Water.—Water is required for—
1. Drinking, washing and bathing.
2. Household purposes like cooking and scrubbing.
3. Town cleaning, especially drains and latrines.
4. Industrial and agricultural purposes.

Quantity Required.—In small towns and villages which have no pipe-line water supply and where people have to carry their water, they find that eight gallons a day is about enough for each member of the family. If the water is brought in pipes near to the houses, much more is used. It has been found that every person in a town uses about twenty-five gallons a day. In an up-to-date town the authorities ought to supply at least thirty gallons of water per day per head of the population. Many towns use 100 gallons per head of the population. Cattle need 10 gallons per head.

SOURCES OF WATER SUPPLY

Rain is the source of all our water. When it falls:

(*a*) Some of it sinks into the ground and forms springs, or is reached by digging wells.

(*b*) Some of it flows downwards and joins a brook, stream or river, and then goes to the sea.

(*c*) Some of it turns into vapour and goes back into the air and will fall again later as rain, hail or snow.

Rain-water is the purest form of water found in nature. It picks up impurities after it falls.

In the tropics, specially where streams and wells are few, we rely greatly on direct rainfall as a source of supply. The rain as it falls is free from disease germs; it is often rendered impure during collection and storage. We shall consider the important question of storage later. Rain is usually collected off the roofs of houses by means of gutters and pipes leading to tanks. The roofs are almost sure to be dirty before the rain falls, and we have to see that the first washings off the roof do not enter the tank. This may be done by turning the delivery pipe by hand away from the tank until the roof has been well washed.

A simple automatic way is to have the gutter perforated; that is, have a hole at the bottom every few inches. The first shower that falls washes the roof and runs through these holes. The rain which follows goes partly through the holes, of course, but plenty runs into the tank. The holes also prevent old and bent gutters from breeding mosquitoes.

Properties of Rain-water.—1. It is soft. That is, it does not contain certain minerals, and will easily make a lather with soap.

2. It easily dissolves lead. This is a disadvantage as lead is rather poisonous. We must be careful not

to allow rain-water to collect in tanks made of lead.
3. It is sparkling because of the air dissolved in it.

GOOD OR BAD SOURCES OF DRINKING WATER

(*a*) Good—
1. Spring water, especially deep springs.
2. Water from deep wells with good walls.

(*b*) Suspicious—
3. Upland surface water (lakes).
4. Stored rain-water.
5. Water from badly built wells.

(*c*) Dangerous—
6. Water flowing through cultivated lands.
7. Rivers which flow through villages and towns.
8. Water from surface wells.

1. Springs.—These, as has already been stated, are
caused by the rain sinking into the soil. The water

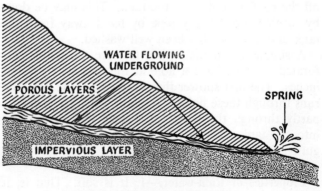

Fig. 9.—Formation of a Surface Spring.

sinks through various porous layers such as earth and
gravel, until it comes to some rock or clay through

which it cannot pass. This is called an Impervious Layer. The water now has to flow the way this layer slopes. In a hilly country the layer may at some place reach the surface, and at this spot the water flows out forming a *surface* spring. In *Deep Springs*, water comes up through a hole in the impervious layer. If such a hole is bored and a pipe put in, the rare form of well called " Artesian " is made. It is really a spring.

Spring water is usually free from impurities and, having air in it, is pleasant to drink.

The hardness of spring water depends on the nature of the soil through which it has passed. If the soil is gravel the water will be soft; if it is chalky the water will be hard because some chalk is dissolved in it.

Medicinal Springs are produced when the soil contains salts which are supposed to be good as medicine.

2. Wells.—As wells are the commonest private source of supply of water it is important to know something about them. Wells are of two kinds Shallow and Deep.

Shallow or Surface Wells.—These are wells which are dug no deeper than the porous layers of the soil. They are the kind commonly seen in our compounds and are usually classified as " dangerous ". The danger is that sewage and rubbish of all kinds may find their way through the soil into the well. This can happen in two ways: (1) Dirt from the surface may soak through the soil in rainy weather and so find its way into the well. (2) Germs from latrines in the neighbourhood may be carried by the flow of underground water into the well especially after heavy rains.

If therefore we have a surface well we must take the following precautions:

1. The land around the well must be kept as clean

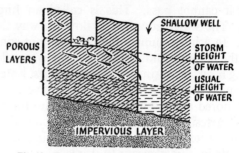

Fig. 10.—Fouling of a Shallow Well after heavy rain.

as possible and, above all, no latrine should be dug nearer than 100 yards from the well.

2. The upper part of the well to a depth of 10–12 feet should be bricked in and rendered water-tight.

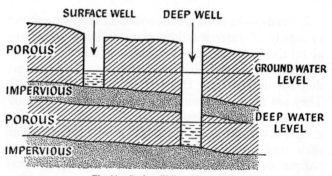

Fig. 11.—Surface Well and Deep Well.

This ensures that water entering the well shall have sunk a good way into the earth. If the water enters the well near the surface, there is a greater danger that it will be unsafe for drinking.

3. The top of the well should have a wall around it and be covered with a good lid. This prevents surface

water from flowing into it and, besides making the
well safe for children and animals, prevents leaves,
dust, manure and so on from falling in.

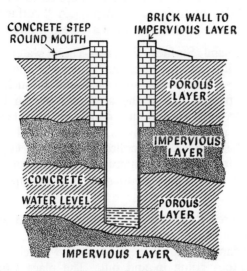

Fig. 12.—A Good Well.

4. The ground immediately around the well should
be cemented, and channels for waste water provided.

5. If possible, a pump should be fitted, as buckets
let down are sure to carry some dirt into the water.

If these conditions are observed a shallow well
is rendered safer, but it is difficult to make it safe from
sewage from near-by latrines and cesspools.

Deep Wells.—These are wells which pass through
the first impervious layer and get to water below it.
They must be cemented or bricked-in all the way to
the first impervious layer, so as not to mix surface and
deep water. The advantage is that all the water here

has travelled a long way underground and is consequently well filtered. They are expensive to make but give good water (see Fig. 12).

Notice that the term " deep " applied to wells gives us no idea of their actual depth. A " surface " well might possibly be deeper than a " deep " one.

3. Upland Surface Waters.—These waters collect from hilly or mountainous districts, and include the lakes, brooks and streams found in such places. If few people live in the area and the land is not cultivated, there is not much danger of the water getting contaminated. Large towns often obtain their water from this source. They collect the water in large lakes (reservoirs) so that the supply during the rainy season will not be wasted, and then carry it by pipes to the town.

4. Stored Rain-water.—(See also pages 23 and 34.) The main dangers are mosquitoes and dirt.

The tank or barrel must have a lid which will stop mosquitoes going in and out. The place where the water runs in must be protected from them by some wire gauze. Protection from dirt is also very important. If the tank has no tap, the dipper should be floating on the water. Hands, cups and pots must not be dipped in it.

5. Water from Cultivated Lands.—As there is certain to be sewage on cultivated lands this kind of water is dangerous. It is the ordinary water found on farms and unfortunately is commonly used by villagers. The ponds are often fouled by people washing in or near them as well as by sewage.

6. Rivers.—One can easily see why rivers are classified as dangerous. So long as they are far from villages or farms they are fairly safe. When they pass through a village they receive the refuse of the houses and, almost certainly, some of the sewage.

Rivers, however, purify themselves a good deal. The fish in them eat up some of the refuse; so do insects of all kinds living in the water. Water plants also aid by giving off oxygen which purifies the organic matter. So great is the effect of these animals and plants, and also of bright sunlight, that a river sometimes completely purifies itself even after receiving the sewage of great cities. All the same, it is not safe to drink unboiled river water, though it may be used for washing.

Impurities in Water.—We have already spoken of certain impurities that water may contain. They may be *Mineral impurities* either dissolved (as in medicinal springs) or suspended (as in muddy water). Or they may be *Organic impurities*. These are more dangerous, and consist of animal or vegetable refuse which gets into the water—(1) by being thrown into a river as it passes a town, (2) by passing from a latrine into wells or rivers, or (3) by a river passing through boggy and marshy land.

Effect of these Impurities.—*Sewage* is the most dangerous as it may contain not only decaying animal and vegetable matter but also germs of disease. The two diseases Typhoid and Cholera are mostly caused by water-borne germs.

Decaying organic matter has a bad effect on the stomach, causing diarrhœa.

Mineral Impurities.—The common mineral impurities are Chalk, Common Salt, Epsom Salts, Glauber's Salts and Lead.

Lead is the most dangerous of these. It may be dissolved from lead pipes, and often produces lead poisoning, which is a serious illness. Copper pipes are best.

Common Salt is often found in water near the sea; a little salt from the sea is harmless. But away from the sea, water which is found to have salt in it usually comes from near a latrine. If that is so, the latrine and the well must be disused for some months. When the water is shown, by special medical tests, to be free from salt and germs, the well may be used.

Epsom and *Glauber's Salts* have no ill-effects. Only small amounts occur in even the strongest natural medicinal water.

Chalk is often found in water, as it is present in many rocks. Its chemical name is *Calcium Carbonate*, and its effect is to make the water hard. Chalk will not dissolve in pure water, but dissolves readily in water which contains carbon dioxide. Now the rain-water which sinks through the soil always absorbs CO_2 from the soil and therefore is able to dissolve chalk from the rocks. Chalky water is safe and pleasant to drink.

HARDNESS OF WATER

Water is said to be *hard* when it is difficult to make it lather with soap. Hardness is due to mineral impurities present. Therefore water which has passed through little soil is likely to be softer. Rain-water is the softest, then come in order upland surface water, river, spring and deep well waters.

The mineral impurities in hard water are harmless to the body, but they spoil the water for washing.

1. Hard water wastes soap, and as soap is expensive this is a disadvantage. The soap has no cleansing power till the scum has stopped forming.

2. The scum formed by the soap interferes with washing and spoils the utensils.

3. Hard water on being boiled deposits "fur", which spoils pots and kettles. This fur is dangerous in engine boilers, as it chokes up the pipes and may cause explosions. One name for it is "kettle-stone".

4. Hard water is not quite so good as soft water for cooking purposes.

The advantages of hard water are:

1. It usually has a pleasant taste.

2. It is not so liable as soft water to dissolve lead and zinc from pipes and tanks.

To Soften Hard Water.—1. Boil the water. This drives off the carbon dioxide and the chalk can no longer remain in the water, which deposits it as fur.

2. For large quantities boiling would be too expensive. So we add quicklime. This lime unites with the carbon dioxide, forming chalk, which falls to the bottom. The water, having no more CO_2 in it, cannot dissolve any chalk; all its chalk falls to the bottom.

If water contains Epsom Salts or Calcium Sulphate, the hardness cannot be removed by boiling. This is called "Permanent Hardness"; the hardness due to chalk is called "Temporary Hardness".

PURIFICATION OF WATER

This is an important subject as impure water causes disease. In the tropics, our supply of water is often from a suspicious or dangerous source. Water may be purified in the following ways.

1. Boiling.—This is one of the best ways, for—

(a) It kills disease germs.

(b) It destroys organic impurities.

The disadvantages connected with it are—

(a) That it takes time and is expensive.
(b) That boiled water is insipid to the taste.
(c) It has to be cooled.

Still, water that has been boiled is the safest for drinking purposes.

To boil every drop of water that we are going to drink is often impossible, but when we are travelling or have newly settled anywhere, it is wise to drink only boiled water. Many people drink only tea in such circumstances. If the only water which can be found is obviously muddy and impure, it must be filtered before boiling.

In places where the water supply is clear, boil the water only in times when water-borne diseases are epidemic (see page 152). Store it in a vessel which has been boiled and fitted with a close-fitting lid.

2. Filtration.—By means of filtration we try to make the water clear and, if possible, free of germs.

Public Filters.—For towns, the water, after being collected from some upland surface, is filtered. The best form of filter is the *Sand filter*. A simple experiment shows how this works. Take a large pot or drum and make a small hole in the bottom. Cover the hole with wire gauze. Now put in some broken-up brick. Next make a layer of gravel and then a layer of sand. This is now a filter, built up like the " waterworks " filters. Pour some muddy water into the pot and after a time it will drop through the hole quite clear.

In public works these filters are very large. The sand requires to be removed and washed from time to time and occasionally renewed. Before the water is poured on, it is stored for some time. It is said that after being stored in the reservoir for four weeks 99 per cent of the disease germs will have been destroyed by sunlight and oxygen. This storing also causes the

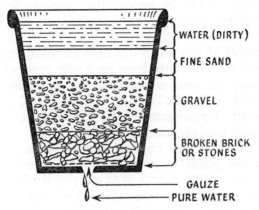

WATER (DIRTY)

FINE SAND

GRAVEL

BROKEN BRICK OR STONES

GAUZE
PURE WATER

Fig. 13.—A simple Sand Filter.

mud to sink to the bottom, and in doing so it drags many germs with it.

Other Methods.—Sometimes other methods are employed, especially where the water is wanted quickly. One method is to add alum to the water. This makes a flaky substance like jelly in the water and when it settles it carries down with it all kinds of mud and germs. In other waterworks the water is mixed with iron salts instead of alum. The effect, as before, is to entangle germs and mud and cause them to sink to the bottom, leaving the water clear.

House Filters.—These remove dirt and germs by passing the water through unglazed pottery in the form of hollow " candles ". They are not so safe as boiling. If the water is very dirty they soon get clogged up and become useless. Germs can stick and multiply in the substance of the filter and infect new water. Filters have to be regularly cleaned, and the candles in them boiled. The water should be boiled after filtering. In fact, house filters are rarely of any use.

Chemical Methods.—In war time, chemical methods of purifying water have been used with great success, and saved the lives of thousands of men. The idea is to add to the water chemicals which kill germs. Potassium Permanganate and Chlorine are two commonly used chemicals.

If the water in the bucket has an unpleasant smell, add a few grains of potassium permanganate. The pink colour will disappear. Add more until a faint pink colour remains. It will be safe to drink half an hour later, but even so, boiling is better and quicker.

Chlorine is used in waterworks where experts are at hand to decide the quantities. Some bleaching powder preparations which produce chlorine are also sold, for purifying water at home or on journeys. Water purified solely by chlorine ought to taste a little sour; if it does not, there is not enough chlorine in it to make it safe. Chlorine needs half an hour to act.

Storage of Water.—In tropical countries people often depend for their supply of water on tanks, especially during the dry season. These tanks are usually filled by collecting the rain as it falls on the roof of the house and carrying it by gutters and pipes. Sometimes the tank is filled by piping water to it from a stream.

The Material of the tank.—Galvanized iron is a good material so long as the zinc coating is intact. No lead should be used in making the tank as rain-water dissolves lead and it might cause lead poisoning. Wooden tanks or barrels are not ideal as wood is liable to rot and spoil the water. Glazed earthenware may be used for storing drinking water.

Sometimes large tanks are made underground. They are lined with cement or tiles and are convenient when large quantities of water are to be stored. These underground tanks have one disadvantage, however: as in the case of surface wells, unless the walls are water-tight, ground water may enter them. On no account should they be near a latrine or cesspit, and care should be taken that they are well covered over.

The tank should be built in a place easily got at, and should be so made that a person can enter it to clean it out. It must have a tightly fitting lid to keep out lizards, insects, etc. All openings should be protected with fine wire gauze to keep out mosquitoes.

The water should be raised from the tank by means of a pump and not by buckets, otherwise dust, leaves and other dirt may get into the tank and foul the water. Needless to say all tanks should be cleaned each year. They also need to be well ventilated to keep them from smelling bad; the air between the water and the top of the tank has to be connected with the outside air by means of wide pipes screened by gauze.

Chapter 5

FOOD

We have considered Air and Water as necessities of the human body, and have seen that without pure air and pure water the body cannot carry on its work.

We now come to another necessity—that of *good food*. We need food for four reasons:

1. To give us Strength.—Food enables us to move and work. We may compare a man with a steam engine and his food with wood or coal. If the stoker does not put fuel on the fire the engine stops. The strength we obtain from food is usually called " energy ".

2. To make us grow.—An underfed child does not grow tall and big. Food is needed to make new bone, new blood, new flesh.

3. To repair our bodies.—Just as an engine gets worn out by constant use, so do our bodies. As we have seen, our breathing and living are like burning. Waste stuff is produced day by day and is thrown off from the body by the excretory system. This waste has to be replaced by food. A man who does not eat soon gets thin and finally dies of starvation.

4. To keep us warm.—We are constantly losing the heat of our bodies. In order to keep alive, our bodies must have a certain amount of heat, and this is obtained from our food. The fuel makes the engine hot as well as making it work, our food gives us warmth as well as energy.

CLASSES OF FOOD

To learn how foods are divided into classes a little knowledge of chemistry is a help. All substances may be divided into two great classes, *Organic* and *Inorganic*. *Organic* substances are obtained from animals or vegetables. *Inorganic* means *mineral:* inorganic foods are *salts* (see p. 40). The Organic Foods are:

(1) Those which contain Nitrogen, the Proteins.
(2) Fats and Oils.
(3) Sugars and Starches, or Carbohydrates.
(4) Vitamins.

Organic Foods containing Nitrogen.—These are called *Proteins.* Their uses are:

(1) To make flesh.
(2) To repair the waste of the body.
(3) They also produce heat and energy.

Some of the chief proteins are:—*Casein* in milk and cheese, *myosin* in lean meat, *legumin* in beans and peas, *albumin* in eggs. *Gelatin,* from bones and gristle, contains nitrogen but is no use to us as protein.

Fats and Oils contains no nitrogen and are sometimes called hydrocarbons. Their uses are:

(1) To warm the body.
(2) To produce energy.
(3) To make fat. Fat serves as a store of food (as, for example, in the hump of a cow or camel) and also protects delicate organs in the body.

Fats and Oils are taken in the body as Butter (85 per cent of this is actual oil and it is very digestible), Cream, Milk, Eggs (11 per cent), various oils (Ground Nut Oil, Coconut Oil, Palm Oil, Olive Oil), Beef and Mutton fat and Pork (about 70 per cent fat).

Sugars and Starches.—These contain carbon but no nitrogen. They contain hydrogen and oxygen in the same proportion as water does and hence are called

D

Carbohydrates. They are a very important group of food-stuffs. Like the Fats and Oils, they:

(1) Warm the body.
(2) Give energy.
(3) Form fat in the body.

As starches and oils do much the same work in the body, one might think that they could be interchanged in our meals. But it is found that this is not the case. We need both fats and carbohydrates, and much more of the latter than of the former. Sugars and starches are cheaper than fats.

Sugar is obtained from the Sugar Cane. *Beet sugar* is identical, and the same sugar is present in honey and Sugar Maple. *Grape Sugar* or *Glucose* comes from fruits, and *Milk Sugar* from the milk of animals. Saccharine is not a kind of sugar but is a harmless flavouring material.

Starch.—Starch is present in most seeds and roots, and is the principal food of man. The starch can be seen under the microscope to be in little balls called starch grains. These balls are hard, but cooking bursts them and sets the starch free. This shows the importance of cooking all starchy foods well before eating. " Pap ", which is prepared by boiling the starch, is a splendid food, as the starch is liberated from the grain so that the digestive juices in the mouth can get to it and make it of use to the body. " Fufu ", made of roots or plantain, well beaten with a heavy pestle after boiling, is also very good; so is " mochi ", made by beating boiled rice with a mallet.

The following are the chief starch foods: Rice, Sweet Potato, Potato, Sago, Tapioca (cassava), Cocoyam or Taro, Yam, Millet, Plantain (cooking banana), Maize, Wheat, Oats.

Vitamins.—When people have all the protein and fat and starch food that they need and plenty of water and the proper salts, you might expect them to grow and to be quite strong. It is found, however, that they suffer from certain sicknesses unless the food they eat includes certain special things. Sailors on ships in the old days used to suffer from *scurvy*. Their gums bled, and blood escaped under the skin, in the bones and elsewhere. A lot of them died. When some lemon-juice was added to their daily food, this disease did not occur.

Again, children fed largely on white bread and margarine made from vegetable oils used to have a disease called *rickets* in their bones, even if lime salts were given to them. Their joints would swell up and be very painful; the bones grew a bad shape. When they had dairy butter or cod liver oil, or when the margarine was improved, their bones grew properly.

A third sickness called *beriberi* comes when people eat little but rice from which the brown part has been removed. If this brown part (rice polishings) is given to them like a medicine they do not get the disease. Beriberi either spoils the nerves or makes the body swell up. Another trouble, *pellagra*, occurs in people who eat little but maize, and causes skin rashes, diarrhoea and mental dullness. It is cured by brewers' yeast.

There must be something in this brown part of the rice or in the lemon-juice or animal oil which is needed by the body. It is the part of food called a *vitamin*. Where can we get enough of these vitamins? We can easily get fruit; we can get rice which has not been milled; we can eat brown bread; we should be able to grow lettuces, red peppers (chillies), tomatoes and green vegetables. Many of us, however, find it difficult to get the right kind of animal fat; we cannot all buy dairy butter. Fortunately, however, we can make this vitamin in our own bodies if we have enough red palm oil or carrots; these contain what the body needs in order to make this vitamin. This it can only do if we are out in the sun enough.

The wheat, rice and maize vitamins are spoken of as Vitamin B. The oil ones are Vitamin A and D. The fruit vitamin is C; it is also found in tomatoes, oranges, lemons, and in the European turnip and swede, as well as in green food which has not been boiled for more than a few minutes. Many other vitamins have been discovered. We need not learn much about them because we get enough of them if we eat plenty of fresh fruit and dairy produce. Poor people often get more vitamins than rich people because they eat more green leaves, chillies, brown rice, and red palm oil. Tinned fruit or jam often has had its vitamins spoiled by heat.

Salt.—Certain kinds of salt are essential to the body:

Common Salt is needed to keep the blood salted, and to form the gastric juice of the stomach which is needed for digesting food.

Lime Salts are necessary to make bone. They are found in milk, eggs and green food, beans and dried fish.

Iron Salts are needed for the red cells of the blood. These salts are found in meal, red meat and green leaves.

Phosphorus is needed for bone, brain and nerves. It is found in most foods, especially in milk, cheese, fish, nuts and cereals.

These and other inorganic salts are not eaten directly, but are found in organic foods. Common salt, however, is also added in cooking and while eating.

We will now consider some of the common articles of food and discuss their value.

ANIMAL FOODS

Red Meat.—Meat gives us most of the proteins we require. About two-thirds of a piece of meat is water, one-third food. This food is two-thirds protein and the rest is fat with a little of each of several salts. Of course in some meat the fat will be greater and the protein less.

Beef is the most nutritious of meats. It is digestible and has less fat than mutton or pork. The flesh is best when the animal is four or five years old.

Mutton.—The flesh of the sheep is finer than goat but both are good.

Pork.—The flesh of the pig is fat but tasty. Pigs are best kept in sties. If allowed to roam about they eat a lot of filth and may spread roundworms and jiggers.

Meat and Tapeworms.—Both beef and pork, even if passed by inspectors at the slaughter house, may contain the young form of worms. If not roasted or grilled right through or if boiled in too large pieces these young worms may not be killed by the heat and can grow to tapeworms in us.

Fish.—Fish forms an important article of diet in coast and river towns. It is more watery than beef but it contains a fair amount of protein. The salts in fish contain phosphorus which enters into the composition of nerves and brain. Some fish, like herring, salmon and eel, have also a good percentage of fat. These *oily fish* are not so good for sick people as white fish, like cod and sole, but are richer in flavour.

Shell-fish, such as crabs and lobsters, must be well cooked. Shell-fish often feed on filth, so they must be thoroughly cleaned and boiled.

All fish are liable to decompose or " go bad " quickly

in tropical climates, so it is important to cook the fish or smoke them over a fire as soon as possible after they are caught.

Poultry.—The flesh of birds, especially the breast, is rich in proteins and is a valuable food. There is usually little fat, and it is easily digested. Birds are generally tender and of good flavour. The tropical village chicken is usually very small, but, with proper methods of poultry-farming, there is no reason why large fowls, ducks, turkeys, etc., giving large eggs and a lot of meat, should not be produced.

Milk.—Cows' and goats' milk is a staple article of food in some countries. In others, only condensed milk can be obtained. Often, this is used as a luxury for adults; it is more needed as a main part of the diet of babies who are not getting their mothers' milk. One of the best things that could happen in the tropics, from a health point of view, would be the development of goat and cattle farming so as to produce a good milk supply.

Milk contains all the kinds of food required by the body, and for babies it is nature's food.

A pint of milk contains about a tablespoonful of cream, another of cheese and still another, or rather more than one, of milk sugar; there are also some lime and other salts and some vitamins. All the rest is water.

Tinned Milk.—Milk preserved in this way is much used, and is a good substitute for fresh milk. To make it, fresh milk is concentrated by evaporation to about one-quarter of its volume. If sweetened it may be kept open a long time, but if unsweetened it should be used quickly after opening as it soon goes bad.

Dried Milk is becoming more and more used as a substitute for fresh milk. The valuable vitamins of the milk are not lost in the process of drying, and the advantages of dried milk are obvious. It is quite free from germs, and does not go bad when opened.

Boiled Milk.—Though milk is such a perfect food, there may be disease germs in it. For this reason it is a good plan to boil milk, especially goat's milk, if obtained fresh. Although some of the good things in the milk are lost by boiling, the advantages of boiling are so great that it should always be done. Boiled milk is quite digestible and all disease germs are killed. It must of course be kept covered till required for use, to keep off flies and dust. Boiled milk will keep good for a longer time than fresh milk.

Cream.—When milk stands for some time the fat rises to the top and forms *cream*. It is a valuable food. The milk which is left is called:

Skimmed Milk.—This is not so nourishing as fresh milk but is very easily digested, and contains a great deal of casein and salts. It must not be used instead of real milk for babies. But dried skimmed milk is valuable for making extra foods for babies which are being weaned, it helps to prevent malnutrition.

Butter.—Fresh butter is one of the best forms of fat. It is obtained from cream by churning, that is, shaking it in a bottle or barrel so that the fat globules run together. Butter is nearly all pure fat; the rest is mainly water.

Cheese.—This almost all protein. It is made by curdling milk and compressing the curd, which consists of casein together with some fats and salts. Cheese is very nutritious but hard to digest, as the fat in it prevents the digestive juices of the stomach from reaching the casein. It is necessary therefore to chew the cheese well, preferably with bread, before swallowing it.

Eggs.—These are very valuable food. They are very rich in nitrogen (protein) and contain all we want in food, except carbohydrates. They are three-quarters water, the rest being about half protein (albumin) and half fat and salts; they contain some vitamins.

The albumin is mainly in the white of the egg and the fat in the yellow part. If albumin is heated it gets hard and indigestible, and so if eggs are boiled hard they are not so nutritious as when lightly boiled.

Eggs go bad because germs pass through the shell and multiply inside. However, eggs will mostly remain good for several weeks, more specially if they have not been washed. They may be placed in a jar of " waterglass " in which they can be kept for months without going bad. Eggs are also regarded as bad if the chick inside has started to grow.

VEGETABLE FOODS

The foods which belong to the vegetable kingdom contain the five classes of constituents needed for the body, but except in nuts, peas and beans the protein element is very small while the starch class is large.

Vegetable foods are divided into the following groups—(1) Cereals, (2) Roots, (3) Green Vegetables, (4) Peas and Beans, (5) Fruits and (6) Nuts.

(1) Cereals.—The chief cereals are Rice, Millet, Maize (or Corn), Wheat and Oats.

Cereals are grains, the seeds of a grass-like plant. Each grain consists of a lump of starch with a small embryo or " germ " at one end. The germ is the living part of the grain (it is not the same as a germ of disease). Around the lump of starch is a layer of protein called the " pericarp ". If the grain is milled or polished by machinery, this layer comes off with the embryo or germ. This is called bran or polishings, and contains nearly all the vitamins.

(a) **Wheat.**—This is the cereal most used by Europeans. It contains a sticky protein which enables the flour to be made into dough.

Brown Bread, wholemeal variety, is made from flour containing the bran. It is very nutritious. Two-thirds of it is starch; the remaining one-third is half water and half protein, with a very little fat and salts. Bran is useful in another way. It leaves a residue in the intestines and thus promotes the action of the bowels.

White Bread is made from flour which does not contain the bran. In the process of milling, the husk and germ of the wheat are removed and the white central part remains. This is rich in starch but poor in protein and vitamins.

Bread is made by mixing flour with water and making the dough thus produced rise. This is usually done by means of yeast. The yeast plant grows and in doing so produces carbon dioxide gas which spreads through the dough and makes it rise. Flour and water can be made to rise by adding chemicals which produce carbon dioxide (baking powder). After the yeast dough has risen a little it is baked. This makes it rise more, and the yeast plant is killed by the heat of the oven.

(b) **Rice.**—Though rice is the most largely used cereal in the world, it is the least nutritious. It contains less

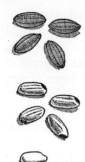

Fig. 14.—Rice Grains:
Top, unhusked;
Middle, husked, but
with germ;
Bottom,   machine
milled, without germ.

protein, fat or salts than most other grains. The starch, however, is easily digested and the protein is of good quality. Rice is usually brown; it is made white by polishing, which removes vitamins and proteins.

(c) **Maize.**—This is a staple food of parts of Asia and Africa. It is a very important and nutritious grain. It cannot be made into bread, but is roasted, or ground into meal. It contains a good deal of fat and the meal cannot be kept long, as it goes sour. Maize is the cereal which approaches nearest in composition to the perfect. But it lacks some things we need, and the absence of these may cause pellagra.

(d) **Millet.**—This name covers a variety of cereal grasses: sorghum; common, Indian, broom-corn or hog millet; fox-tail, pearl, barn-yard and finger millet. It can grow in drier places than most other crops. It is a good food but lacks Vitamin C; green vegetables should therefore be eaten with it. Like other cereals it is poor in protein.

(e) **Oats.**—Oatmeal porridge is one of the most nutritious cereal foods, containing a good deal of protein and some fat. It is not good for tiny children.

(2) Roots, Tubers, Plantains and Breadfruit.—These give many of us our chief supply of starch and sugar and do not contain much protein. They are about three-quarters water and one-quarter starch; protein, fats and vitamins occur in them in very small quantities, but they contain a fair amount of useful salts.

The starch is very nutritious, but one cannot live on roots and plantains only as there is not enough protein and fat. It is important to notice that in these roots and tubers most of the protein is situated just beneath the skin, and hence they ought to be cooked in their skins, and peeled afterwards or not at all.

(*a*) **Cassava** or **Tapioca.**—This tuber is the usual food of large numbers of people and is very good starch food, but it contains very little protein. There are two main varieties, the bitter and the sweet. The former, as is well known to the people who use it, is poisonous unless it is properly prepared; when the juice is strained out after grating (garri), or washed away, it is safe. *Sweet Cassava* is so named because it is good to eat after simple baking or frying; it makes good pounded food (fufu); its leaves are edible. The tuber of this plant gives us tapioca.

(*b*) **Yam.**—The best yams are the finest roots in the world to eat; they are also the largest. They are an expensive food to send from place to place, so that they are mainly used near to the countries which grow them. Fufu is the best cooked form of yam.

(*c*) **Plantains.**—These belong to the banana family, but can be eaten boiled before they are ripe. Thus they are eaten while still starchy, whereas a lot of the starch in bananas turns into sugar. Plantains are eaten with soup, like root foods, and are a good food. Many people live on them for months at a time. They also make good fufu.

(*d*) **Cocoyam** or **Taro.**—This is eaten boiled or beaten into fufu. Its leaves are a useful green vegetable.

(*e*) **Sweet Potato.**—This is quite a good starch food. Its leaves are also eaten; they contain calcium and vitamins.

(*f*) **Potato.**—Potatoes are well known but not much grown in the tropics. They are about as good as yams, but their leaves are poisonous.

(*g*) **Breadfruit.**—The fruit of this tree is a very good carbohydrate food. Breadfruit can be either baked or boiled. The taste reminds Europeans of chestnuts; these, however, have more protein than breadfruit. So does the tropical chestnut; but this is so rare that it cannot be regarded as an important food. Curiously enough, the seeds of the breadfruit are also contained in nuts. The flesh around them and the nuts themselves are both good food. Cultivated breadfruit has few or no nuts.

Other roots, such as the turnip, parsnip, carrot, and especially the beet, are valuable on account of their sugar and mineral salts, as well as for vitamins.

(3) Vegetables.—This group of foods covers cabbage, sweet potato leaves and other forms of spinach, pumpkin, tomatoes, and onions; and cucumber and lettuce which are eaten raw as salad. Most of them are valuable on account of the vitamins they contain. They also contain a lot of water, cellulose (the substance composing the cell-walls of plants) and mineral salts. They have little food value but act as a kind of medicine, keeping the body in good order. They are pleasant in taste, and flavour our food and soups. The cellulose tends to prevent constipation.

Caution.—In the tropics it is unsafe to eat vegetables raw for fear of dysentery, cholera and typhoid. Also eggs of various worms may get into the body through them. Vegetables are often grown under very insanitary conditions and are difficult to clean. Cooked vegetables are quite safe and a great aid to health.

(4) Peas and Beans.—The characteristic of the group is the great amount of protein which they contain. They contain Vitamin B. If allowed to sprout, they produce Vitamin C.

They are a valuable flesh-forming food and can take the place of meat in our diet. Very good soups are made with them. Bean pudding or cake is made by frying pounded beans with oil or fat, and forms a very nutritious food.

(5) Fruits.—Fruits are liked for their taste but care must be taken that they are not rotten, and also that the skins, if they are eaten, are clean. Some fruits are good as food, such as *grapes* (containing much sugar), and *dates* (which contain starch and sugar). *Bananas* and *breadfruit* also contain starch and are foods. Besides being valuable for their vitamins, fruits are useful as laxatives.

Pawpaw or *papaya* is a fruit or a vegetable. Its leaves contain a ferment which aids in the digestion of meat. It can be eaten ripe as a fruit or boiled when green and eaten as a vegetable.

(6) Nuts.—These are useful as supplying protein and especially fat. Nuts can be grated into a fine powder and thus made more digestible. The tropics are rich in nuts which yield oils that are used to make food-stuffs, for example, coconut, palm nut, ground nut (peanut), which is really a bean, and shea butter.

CONDIMENTS

Condiments are used in order to add flavour and taste to our food. They are not foods themselves. They promote the flow of digestive juices and so stimulate digestion. They are like the whip to a horse, which must not be used in excess or the horse will get tired. An excessive use of condiments will do harm to the digestion. The chief condiments are pepper, mustard, vinegar, ginger and cloves. Red peppers or chillies are strong stimulants and contain Vitamin C.

TINNED FOODS

The principle underlying the tinning or canning of foods is that germless food cannot decay; so that all kinds of food, meat, vegetables, fish, fruit or milk, when enclosed in air-tight tins, can keep good for an indefinite time. Obviously this offers great advantages. Countries which produce an excess of fruit need not waste it, but may send it to less fortunate parts of the world in tins. So also with any other food. Travellers can be sure of a supply of good food, and people living in a foreign land can still get their native dishes.

Again, many fruits are seasonal; when they are tinned, it is possible to have fruit to eat all the year round.

Tinned foods may, however—

(1) Lose some of their food value, especially vitamins, in the process of tinning.

(2) Contain germs which make the contents poisonous. Therefore—

(1) See that the tin does not bulge. Germs produce gas which blows out the tin.

(2) The tin should not be rusted or dented. The ends, however, should be slightly hollow.

When the tin has been opened turn the contents out

into a dish, otherwise poisons may be formed by the food touching the tin in the presence of the air. This rule is very important, unless the tins are of first-class quality or the food contains sugar or other preservative.

Chapter 6

BEVERAGES OR DRINKS

Beverages are used (1) to supply in an agreeable form a great deal of the water needed by the body; (2) to provide extra food and vitamins; and (3) as a matter of custom on social occasions.

The chief beverages in use all over the world are tea, coffee and cocoa; beers, wines and spirits; and fruit juices.

Let us briefly study these in order.

TEA

Tea consists of the dried leaves of a plant and was introduced by the Chinese; it has found its way to every part of the world. It is grown in India and Ceylon, and lately in Africa.

To make Tea.—Make the pot hot by pouring in boiling water. When the pot is hot pour the water out. Then put the tea into this pot—one teaspoonful for each pint or so—and pour *boiling* water on it; the water *must be actually boiling* when poured on the tea. Allow it to stand for three minutes, when it is ready to drink. Made in this way it will contain everything of value in the tea and nothing that is harmful. Beware of " Bush teas ", they are often harmful.

Advantages of Tea as a Beverage.—1. It ensures that the water taken into the body has been boiled and is thus free from germs.

2. It stimulates the heart's action and quickens the breathing. Thus it acts as a stimulant.

3. By causing perspiration it cools the body.

4. It can warm the body if taken hot. Hot sweet tea is excellent for shock.

Disadvantages.—Tea has no disadvantages if it is properly made and taken in moderation. But—

1. If tea is boiled or left too long in contact with the leaves, a substance called *tannin* comes from them which gives the tea a bitter taste and does harm.

2. If strong tea is taken in excess it has a bad effect on the digestion and nerves.

COFFEE

Coffee is the berry of a plant grown originally in Arabia and now in many parts of Asia and Africa. The dried beans are roasted and this develops the flavour. The roasted beans are ground and are then ready for use. The coffee should, if possible, be freshly ground so as to retain the full flavour.

Coffee powder makes an excellent drink, and bottled coffees are quite harmless.

Coffee compared with Tea.—1. It is also a stimulant but is more powerful.

2. Taken in excess it produces the same effects as tea, but in addition it causes sleeplessness.

Special use of Coffee.—Strong coffee will counteract some of the poisonous effects of alcohol and opium.

To make Coffee.—A special coffee-pot consists of two parts, upper and lower. The upper part has a perforated bottom, and fits over the lower.

Freshly roasted and ground coffee is put in the upper part and covered with boiling water. The coffee strains through into the bottom part. Coffee may be made like tea or even boiled in a pan.

Chicory is often mixed with coffee. It is a bitter-tasting root which is dried, roasted and ground before use. Some think it brings out the flavour of the coffee.

COCOA

Cocoa contains a considerable amount of fats, proteins and starch, and is therefore a food as well as a stimulant.

Cocoa comes from the cocoa tree which is widely grown in West Africa. The beans and some of the jelly that surrounds them are taken from the pod, allowed to ferment and dried in the sun or over a fire. They may then be sent to a factory to be made into tinned cocoa. Or they can be pounded into a paste, rolled into sticks and left to cool and harden. The sticks are grated before use; this powder needs boiling in water, then it is best to cool it, skim off the surface fat and heat it again. Tinned cocoa can be made into a drink by pouring boiling water on to it, stirring it all the time; but actual boiling improves it. Add sugar and milk.

BEERS, WINES AND SPIRITS

Alcohol enters into the composition of a great many beverages and is present in palm wine, toddy and other home-made fermented drinks. It is produced by the fermentation of sugar when *yeast* is added; this acts upon the sugar, producing alcohol and carbon dioxide.

Alcoholic drinks vary greatly in their nature and

E

strength. *Beers* and *Ales*, made from hops and malt, have from 2 to 12 per cent of alcohol. *Wines* contain up to 20 per cent of alcohol. They are obtained by fermenting grape juice.

Spirits.—These are produced by distilling other alcoholic liquors and are merely alcohol diluted with water and flavoured. They may contain over 50 per cent of alcohol. During distillation, some other things are produced. Cheap rum, gin, whisky and brandy still contain these by-products. As some of them, called Fusel Oils, are poisonous, they are removed from " high-class " spirits.

Effects of Alcohol.—Alcohol has many effects upon the body. The following are a few:

1. It numbs the nervous system.
2. It causes the blood-vessels to dilate.
3. It increases the heart-beat for a time.
4. In the long run, it harms the stomach and liver.

When taken with food, alcohol has little effect on digestion; taken on an empty stomach, it impairs digestion, particularly of Vitamin B. Though it gives the sensation of warmth, it really lowers the temperature of the body and is therefore dangerous in cases of exposure to cold.

It is, however, on the nervous system that alcohol has its worst effect. It poisons the higher brain and nerve centres, blunts the sensibilities and interferes with the power of judgment. It hinders one from doing fine and delicate work with one's hands, because the control of the muscles is affected. This is specially true of drivers; decisions have to be made and acted upon very quickly when driving, and even the delayed decision caused by palm wine often causes a serious accident. Unfortunately, too, a driver who has had a drink or two usually thinks he is driving better.

Judgment in moral matters is spoiled in the same way. Men and women often catch venereal diseases from each other when they have been drinking. There is no danger, however, of disease germs in the actual drink; alcohol kills most of the germs.

Alcohol was thought to be a food, but it has little food value. It is also said to be a stimulant, but other stimulants are better. It may soothe nerves and allay anxiety. Many scientific men advise that it should never be used as a beverage, and in view of its bad effects, every civilized government has laws to limit its use; the Mohammedan religion forbids it entirely.

FRUIT DRINKS

Orange juice, which is a pleasant drink with or without extra sugar and water, is rich in Vitamin C; so are pineapple and tomato juice. Fruit drinks are valuable too; but many bottled soft drinks simply consist of water with tasty chemicals and carbon dioxide. They have little food value. They are harmless if they contain no disease germs. Mineral water factories must have high standards of cleanliness.

The Siamese villager uses coconut " milk " as a drink to welcome a visitor. It is the world's best beverage.

PALM WINE

Palm wine, when fresh, is a healthy drink and contains a lot of Vitamin B. But many people prefer to keep it until it ferments and produces alcohol, when it diminishes self-control, makes one merry, then drunk.

Chapter 7

DIET AND COOKING

We have considered the chief foods and beverages but there still remains the question of how these should be taken in our meals. We know that a man could not live by eating nothing but yam, even if he had an unlimited quantity. We have learnt that we require the following classes of food: Proteins (nitrogen foods), Carbohydrates (sugar and starch), Fats, Vitamins and various kinds of Salt.

Nature's food for growing children, milk, contains all these classes in the proportions required; but for full-grown men and women the quantities and proportions required are found by appetite and taste.

We lose substance from our bodies by excretion through the bowels, kidneys, lungs and skin; this loss ought to be just equal to what we take in as food.

It is found that one-sixth part of all the food we take ought to be protein.

When we come to actual articles of food, however—bread, meat, oils and so on—we find that in any one food the ratio of protein to starch is not what we require. By eating bread only, we may get enough protein if we eat a large quantity, but in doing so we shall overstock our bodies with carbohydrates.

If we were to eat just enough bread to get the carbohydrate right, and nothing else, we should not get sufficient protein to keep us in health.

A MIXED DIET

As foods do not contain the correct proportions of starch, protein and fat, we have to mix them. As a matter of fact, no one would like to eat nothing but rice or nothing but yam. We naturally take soup with it. The soup contains oil, vegetables, peppers and meat. These have fats, salts, vitamins and proteins, but practically no starch.

Another good mixture is pap—a sort of thick gruel—and bean pudding. The pap is mainly starch, and the bean pudding contains oil, salts, condiments and also a lot of protein. Plantains fried in oil also give a fair mixture, though deficient in protein.

Of European foods the following give us the food classes in good proportions: potatoes and meat; bread and cheese; pork and beans; curry and rice.

OVER-FEEDING AND UNDER-FEEDING

Even if the food we eat has the correct proportions, our meals may be wrong through being too large or too little.

Over-feeding.—When the appetite is satisfied no more food should be eaten however attractive it may be. The digestive system can only manage a certain amount of food; food in excess stays in the intestines too long undigested. This food may ferment, causing wind and perhaps constipation.

Under-feeding.—A person who eats too little becomes thin and weak and is less able to resist disease than a properly fed man. Especially is he liable to get fever, tuberculosis and infectious diseases, and if he already has some disease he will be made worse by under-feeding.

Protein lack.—This is common in many tropical areas where meat, fish and eggs are scarce and people eat too much starchy food. Children get thin, with a pale skin which peels off, and their hair goes brown or reddish and loses its curls. Later the belly swells and the face gets puffy. Some call this *kwashiorkor* but doctors know it as protein malnutrition, and it can be cured by milk protein and prevented by good vegetable protein from beans and ground nuts when meat is scarce.

Times of Meals.—This is a more important question than it seems. The best plan is to have three meals a day, say at 7 a.m., midday and 6 p.m., but times must be made to suit the hours of work. The great thing is that meals should be taken regularly at the same hours every day. One of the chief causes of constipation is irregularity of meal-times. The organs of digestion form habits just as do other organs of the body, and they work much better when food is taken at the same times day by day.

Another rule is that food should not be eaten between meals. The reason for this will easily be seen when we study the process of digestion. It is not good for fresh food to be sent down to the stomach when the previous meal is only half digested. The stomach and intestines need rest and should not be made to work continuously.

Some Rules concerning Meals—
1. Eat at regular times.
2. Do not eat between meals.
3. Do not do hard work or take a hot bath just after a meal. The stomach wants the blood which would go to the muscle or the skin.
4. Do not drink much at meals. It is a very good thing, however, to drink plenty of water in the early morning.

5. Rest, or even sleep for half an hour, after a heavy lunch, but do not eat just before going to bed for the night. Both sleep and digestion are disturbed by this.

COOKING

We may conclude the subject of " Food " by considering some of the ways in which food is prepared for eating. There are many reasons why food should be cooked and the subject is important. Bad cooking can render even good food of little value; good cooking can make even poor food attractive. In the tropics there is need for more attention to be given to cooking. There are so many excellent ways of cooking known to the women that it is a pity when people go on eating similar dishes day after day.

The uses of cooking are—
1. To render food more digestible, (*a*) By breaking up starch cells, (*b*) By softening it and helping the teeth in their work of tearing and grinding it, (*c*) By making the food attractive in smell and taste, causing the digestive juices to flow freely, and so aiding digestion, and (*d*) By improving the appetite.
2. Some food such as meat will keep good longer if cooked. This is of great advantage in the tropics.
3. Cooking will kill germs which may happen to be in the food.

Note, however, that cooking diminishes the amount of Vitamin C in the food.

Methods of Cooking Meat and Fish.—These are Boiling, Frying, Stewing and Baking.

1. Boiling.—Boiling makes meat very digestible and most of the meat juices are retained. The flavour, however, is not so good as in the case of baking. To keep the juices inside the meat: (1) The whole joint of meat is plunged into boiling water; this hardens the outside and prevents the escape of the juices. (2) It is then, after say five minutes, allowed to simmer till ready. This takes about twenty minutes for each pound of meat, or an hour for a three-pound joint. Fish cooks in a few minutes.

2. Frying.—A common method of cooking meat, fish, eggs and some vegetables is to fry them in oil or fat. The temperature of boiling oil is much higher than boiling water, so frying is a quick method of cooking. Unless the meat is in thin slices, however, the heat does not reach the centre, and embryo worms or germs may remain alive. This danger exists, in fact, with every method of cooking meat except stewing. That is why pork, the most dangerous meat for worms and germs, should be stewed. Fried foods are hard to digest and should not be taken at every meal, or by invalids or little children.

3. Stewing.—This method is something like boiling but here the object is to have nutriment in both the meat and water. There is therefore no waste. It is the most economical way of cooking. The meat is cut up into small pieces and put in the pot. Often vegetables and condiments are added. A very tasty stew is made by frying the ingredients before stewing. Just sufficient water to cover the contents is added and the whole is heated just to boiling point for some hours. The stew must not be allowed to boil or the meat will get tough. Stewing is suitable for poor meat, tough joints and pork.

If the pork is not from an inspected slaughter-house, it should be boiled in quite small pieces.

4. Baking.—The meat is placed in a dish and then put into an oven. The process is much the same as roasting, an old-fashioned method in which the joint was made to turn round and round in front of the fire. Fat is poured on it from time to time (basting). The oven is first made very hot to harden the surface of the meat, which is then allowed to bake at less heat until cooked. The oven must be ventilated or the meat will not taste its best.

The Dutch oven is a useful kind: it consists of an iron dish half covered by a curved iron hood. This hood can be moved to reflect the heat of the fire on to either side of the meat in the dish. This oven is placed in front of the fire and air can get to the meat, thus avoiding the disadvantages of a closed oven.

The *Haybox* or fuelless cooker: if you fill a box or carton with dry grass, and make a nest inside it to hold a cooking pot or saucepan, you only need to bring the food to the boil and put it into this haybox. It will then keep hot for 3 or 4 hours, long enough to complete the cooking of root foods or a stew with meat in it. The lid of the haybox should have a cushion of hay attached to it inside; a piece of sack-cloth nailed over the hay is enough. This system saves fuel and is most valuable where firewood is scarce. Every school in those areas should have one to demonstrate to the hygiene and cookery classes, and keep it in use. Haybox cooking is very attractive, as food does not become overcooked and too soft. It remains surprisingly hot for a long time.

Vegetables.—The main object in cooking vegetables is to soften the tissues of the green ones, and to break

down the cell walls of those containing starch. Some
vegetables, such as lettuce, cucumber, tomato, radish,
yam bean, Chinese radish, mustard and cress, can be
eaten raw. They must be carefully washed; in times
of typhoid, cholera or dysentery, avoid them (see page
155). The skin and seeds of cucumbers and tomatoes
are edible. Uncooked food is specially good vitamin
food.

Green Vegetables are best cooked in soft water.

To retain their Vitamin C, greens should be dropped
into *boiling* water and cooked for a few minutes only.
Gradual heating destroys the vitamins. Greens water—
except from some cassava leaves—is good to drink or
as part of soup.

Cleanliness in Cooking.—Cleanliness is necessary in
all parts of a house but nowhere more than in the
kitchen. A dirty kitchen is a source of great danger.
Flies and other insects always abound where scraps of
food are left about, and flies carry disease.

Kitchen utensils, pots, pans, spoons and dishes
should always be cleaned immediately after use. The
work of cleaning pans is much harder once the food
has hardened on to them. Grease can best be got off
with hot water and soda or soap; a supply of these
should always be kept in the kitchen.

One of the best metals for kitchen utensils is better-
class aluminium, and with care these can be kept bright,
but soda should not be used. In no case should leaden
or copper vesels be used for cooking.

The *meat safe* should be kept in good repair and no
food should be left uncovered. If a safe is not available,
satisfactory coverings can be made by spreading a
piece of muslin or mosquito netting over a bamboo
frame. Refrigerators are the best way of keeping food

fresh, though they are expensive to buy and to keep going. They should always be emptied and cleaned every week.

Ants are a great nuisance in most hot climates. Sugar and a number of other foods can be kept in tins with a press-on lid. Safes should be made ant-proof where possible; some have legs or hanging devices which ants cannot cross. Placing the legs of a safe in tins of water is good so long as steps are taken to prevent mosquito larvae from breeding in them; either the water must be changed twice a week or it must be covered with a thin film of kerosene. Insecticides (see p. 138) often clear a room of ants.

SECTION II

PHYSIOLOGY

Chapter 8

RESPIRATION

We have studied how to provide good air, water and food, and now we must learn how these are taken into the body and used by it. In the Introduction we saw that the body is organized into the Respiratory, Circulatory, Digestive, Excretory, Nervous and Reproductive Systems. We will now consider these in order.

THE RESPIRATORY SYSTEM

This System is composed of the lungs and the passages leading to them. The object of breathing is to bring the oxygen of the air into contact with the blood and by this means to—

1. Give some oxygen to the blood.
2. Take up waste products from the blood.

The breathing organs are in the chest. They are enclosed in a kind of cage formed by the ribs, the breast-bone and back-bone; the floor of this cage consists of the diaphragm, which is a large sheet of muscle dividing the chest from the abdomen.

The air, in passing to the lungs, has to go through various passages:

The Nose and Mouth.—It is of importance to use the nose and not the mouth for most of our breathing.

When we breathe through the mouth the air passes directly to the back of the throat. When we breathe

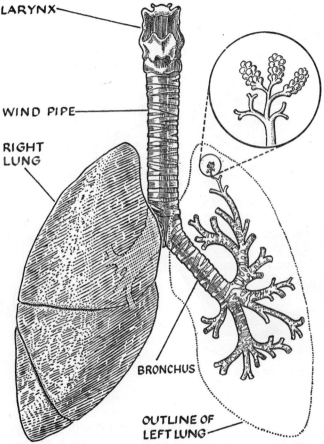

LARYNX

WIND PIPE

RIGHT LUNG

BRONCHUS

OUTLINE OF LEFT LUNG

Fig. 15.—Air passages and lungs. The part shown within the circle is enlarged in Fig. 16.

through the nose the air has to pass through narrow slits and over specially shaped bones which purify and warm the air. The small hairs in the nose are moist and sticky, and prevent dust from reaching the back of the throat. Those who always breathe through the mouth are apt to get sore throat, and possibly tuberculosis and other diseases. Children who cannot breathe

SECTION OUTSIDE VIEW

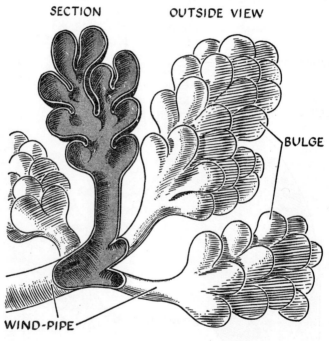

BULGE

WIND-PIPE

Fig. 16.—Showing the air bag in which the wind-pipe ends.

through their noses must be seen by a doctor. It may be due to swellings of the glands at the back of the throat called tonsils and adenoids. These are bad for a child. Doctors can remove them by a small operation.

There are two passages leading downwards from the

nose and mouth into the body, one to take food and water to the stomach, the other to take air to the lungs.

The gullet, or œsophagus, has soft walls and is closed unless food is being swallowed. It is behind the wind-pipe.

The wind-pipe, or trachea, has walls of gristle to keep it from being flattened. At the moment of swallowing the upper end is closed. It can be felt rising up as it closes.

The Larynx or Voice Box.—This is quite easily felt in the throat and is commonly known as " Adam's Apple ". The rest of the wind-pipe is about four inches long and one inch wide. It has from sixteen to twenty rings of gristle which keep it open. It is lined with a smooth shiny skin which has a lot of short " hairs ". These hairs move and sweep any phlegm towards the mouth, where it can be spat into a handkerchief or swallowed.

The wind-pipe at the lower end, divides into two branches, or bronchi, which go to the two lungs. There they divide into a very large number of tubes, getting smaller and smaller till they cannot be seen with the naked eye.

The Lungs are made up of thousands of little air bags called air-sacs, which are really the ends of the smallest wind-pipes. The air-sac is not smooth like a toy balloon, but has many " bulges " on it, and thus has a great amount of surface.

These thousands of air-sacs form the lungs. It is important to understand the structure of these sacs. Around each sac are fine blood-vessels. The walls of the " bulge " and of the blood-vessels are of course extremely thin, and so the blood is almost in contact with the air in the bag.

Most people have seen sheep's lungs. They are

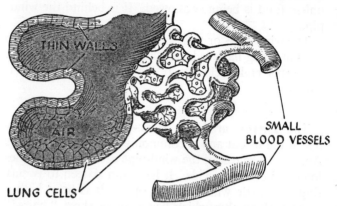

THIN WALLS

AIR

SMALL
BLOOD VESSELS

LUNG CELLS

Fig. 17.—How the blood meets the air in the air-sacs.

spongy to the touch and are very light. They float in water.

The outside of the lungs is covered with a shiny skin called the *Pleura*. If this gets inflamed the person suffers from pleurisy.

The lungs completely fill the chest; there is no air between them and the chest wall. To fill the lungs with air, the chest is made bigger, the lungs expand and the air from outside is sucked into them.

BREATHING

Breathing is made up of Inspiration and Expiration.

Inspiration.—Breathing in is done by enlarging the chest. This is done in two ways:

1. By pulling the chest floor (*Diaphragm*) downwards.
2. By raising the ribs, thus enlarging the sides of the chest.

Usually both these methods of breathing are employed at the same time.

By contraction the diaphragm gets shorter and this

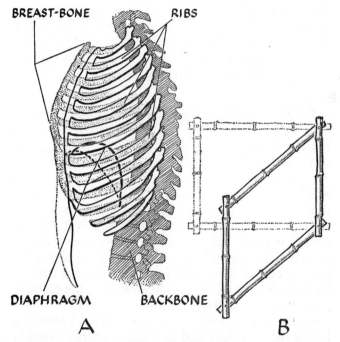

BREAST-BONE   RIBS

DIAPHRAGM   BACKBONE
A   B

Fig. 18a.—Movement of Chest and Diaphragm during inspiration. Dotted lines show ribs raised and diaphragm pulled down.

Fig. 18b.—The area enclosed by these sticks is much larger when the slanting ones are raised. In the same way the chest is much bigger when the ribs are raised.

pulls it down into a lower position. Also the breast-bone and ribs are raised by their special muscles. The effect is to enlarge the chest.

It is found that men and children make more use of the diaphragm in breathing, while women use the ribs more than the diaphragm.

F

Expiration.—Breathing out is done by making the chest smaller. In ordinary expiration the weight of the ribs and the tendency of the lungs to get to their natural size (*elasticity*) are sufficient to do this once the muscles are relaxed. In coughing, whistling, blowing the nose or shouting, more air than usual is expelled. This is done by the diaphragm being pushed farther up into the chest, thus squeezing the lungs and forcing out the air. This is called *forced expiration*.

What happens in the Air-Sacs.—This is where the lung does its work. It is there that the air gets very close to the blood. This blood comes from the body by way of the heart, and is impure. It comes in the *Pulmonary Artery*, which divides into thousands of little vessels, which, by clinging round an air-sac, get very close to the air of the lung. The impure blood is dark red in colour and has too much carbon dioxide in it and not enough oxygen. The wall of the air bag is so thin that gases can pass through it, and an exchange of gases takes place. Some of the oxygen from the air passes into the blood and some of the carbon dioxide of the blood is given to the air in the bag.

As the impure blood receives oxygen it becomes a bright red in colour and is called " arterial blood ". It goes back to the heart and is ready to do its work again.

The new oxygen is taken by the blood all over the body. The muscles need it to do their work and, while doing it, keep the body warm.

Practical Lessons.—From our consideration of the Respiratory System we have learned one or two things of great importance to health. It is one thing to have a good supply of fresh air by ventilation, it is another thing to get this good air into the lungs.

1. We should breathe through the nose and not the mouth whenever possible.

2. We should try to increase the size of the chest and so get larger lungs. This is specially important while we are young. It may be done by (*a*) taking proper exercises which expand the chest and strengthen its muscles, (*b*) breathing deeply and so filling the lungs full now and then, and (*c*) walking, standing and sitting in correct attitudes with the shoulders well back.

3. We should try to avoid chills, which cause phlegm to form in the air passages and lungs, and so hinder the air from entering, and allow germs to grow.

Smoking.—In a book which is to help people to avoid disease, we must look at the diseases which smoking seems either to cause or make worse. The smoking of large numbers of cigarettes is known to cause a big increase in lung disease. Smaller risks are run by cigar and pipe smokers or those who smoke only a few cigarettes. One of these diseases is cancer of the air passages. It is very hard to cure; most people who have it die of it. Another is chronic bronchitis which makes people cough very badly but may not kill them. Smoking may increase tuberculosis of the lungs. It also leads to some forms of heart disease and to indigestion.

People should look at smoking in this way. The more non-smokers there are, the easier it is for others not to smoke. If all of a school of 600 boys become heavy cigarette smokers, 100 will probably die of that lung cancer. If none of them smoked, 85 of those 100 men would be saved from that disease. Every boy who does not smoke and so helps others not to, is saving lives: perhaps his own, certainly someone else's.

Now that women are smoking a lot of cigarettes, they too have more and more lung cancers, so the same advice is good for schoolgirls. Make sure that you develop habits which help you and other people to keep healthy.

Chapter 9

THE BLOOD AND ITS CIRCULATION

The Circulatory System is the means by which the blood gets round the body.

Composition.—Blood is made up of a clear fluid and a great number of solid bodies called *Corpuscles* or *Cells*. The name of the fluid is *Plasma*. When blood is exposed to air it begins to form a clot out of which there comes a pale yellow liquid called *Serum*. After the serum separates from the clot, *Fibrin* (a protein substance) is left in which are entangled all the corpuscles. So we may make a table giving the composition of blood:

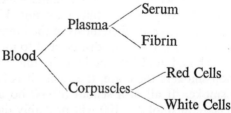

Ordinary blood-clot is fibrin mixed with cells.

The Corpuscles.—There are two kinds, red and white. They are very small cells: there are half a million in a

speck of blood as small as the head of a small pin.
About a thousand of these would be white corpuscles.

Red Corpuscles.—These are discs, shaped like a
small coin but hollowed out on both sides. They
are usually seen piled together like a heap of coins.
Their chief work is to carry a substance called *Hæmoglobin* which is a protein containing a little iron. This
hæmoglobin combines with oxygen to form a bright
red substance which easily loses its oxygen. With
carbon dioxide, on the other hand, hæmoglobin forms
a bluish compound.

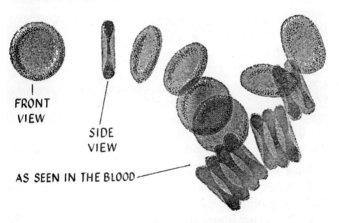

FRONT
VIEW

SIDE
VIEW

AS SEEN IN THE BLOOD

Fig. 19.—Red Blood Corpuscles (Highly magnified.)

It is in this way and not as gases that oxygen and
carbon dioxide are carried about the body. This
explains the change of colour from dark to bright
red when the blood passes through the lungs.

Anæmia.—After severe bleeding, malaria or hookworm and some other diseases, there are too few

red cells to carry the necessary oxygen. This is called *anæmia*. Besides being pale, an anæmic person feels short of breath, especially after making any effort.

White Corpuscles.—These are so-called soldiers or scavengers—and are of great importance. Each is a small jelly-like creature with a *nucleus*, or kernel.

They eat up disease germs which enter the body. These corpuscles eat things by moving towards them and gradually flowing over them (see Fig. 20).

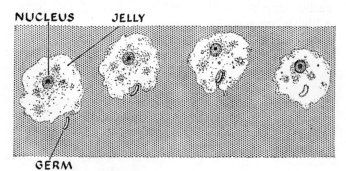

NUCLEUS   JELLY

GERM

Fig. 20.—A White Corpuscle attacking and eating a Germ. (Highly magnified.)

Uses of Blood.—Blood is the carrier of the body.

1. As explained above, it carries oxygen (joined on to hæmoglobin) to parts needing it.

2. It carries impurities from all parts of the body to the skin, kidneys and lungs which get rid of them.

3. It carries food from the digestive organs to the tissues.

4. It cools the parts of the body which are hotter than it is, and warms those which are cooler.

THE CIRCULATION OF THE BLOOD

We have now to find out how the blood is sent round the body. It is only since the time of William

Harvey, an English doctor who died in the year 1657, that it has been known that the blood circulates. Before his time, though the pulse and the heart-beat were known, it was thought the blood went backwards and forwards in the veins. One or two well-known facts prove to us that the blood circulates.

1. If we cut an artery the blood spurts out and these spurts correspond with the heart-beats.

2. If poison gets into, say, a finger, or medicine into a vein, it is soon to be found all over the body.

3. Blood is found in two quite distinct kinds of tubes which are connected with the heart. In one set (veins) it can flow only in one direction because they have valves which will open only one way.

These are only a few of many proofs that the blood flows. With a strong lens one can actually see the blood flowing in the web of a frog's foot.

THE HEART

The heart is a strong muscular organ which acts as the pumping station for the circulation. It is situated in the chest between the right and left lungs and is enclosed in a double bag. It lies behind the breast-bone and the ribs on the left.

Structure.—The heart is divided into two chief rooms by a wall running from top to bottom, the rooms being left and right of this; there is no direct connexion between them. These rooms are themselves divided into two parts, upper and lower, but these parts have doors (valves) between them. The diagram will make this clear. The upper rooms are called *Auricles* and the lower *Ventricles*. The walls of these rooms are made of muscle and are very strong, especially those of the left ventricle.

The Heart at Work.—We will now follow the course of some blood starting from the *Left Ventricle*. Here the blood is bright red and pure, ready to start on its

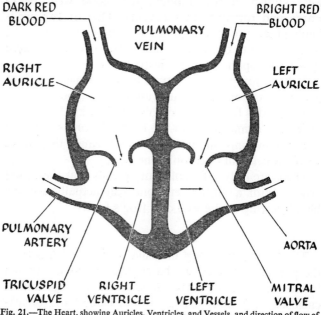

DARK RED BLOOD

BRIGHT RED BLOOD

PULMONARY VEIN

RIGHT AURICLE

LEFT AURICLE

PULMONARY ARTERY

AORTA

TRICUSPID VALVE

RIGHT VENTRICLE

LEFT VENTRICLE

MITRAL VALVE

Fig. 21.—The Heart, showing Auricles, Ventricles, and Vessels, and direction of flow of blood.

journey through the body. Let us suppose the heart commences to beat. A beat consists of two parts:

1. The two auricles are squeezed.
2. Then the two ventricles are squeezed.

When the ventricles squeeze the blood, it presses towards the doors into the auricles. These doors, however, at once close and will not allow the blood to pass that way. On the left side, this door is called the *Mitral Valve*. So the blood now has to escape through the other tube which leads from the left ventricle, called the *Aorta*. This is the largest artery in the body. Where it leaves the left ventricle there is a valve which allows blood to flow only from the heart into the aorta and not back again into the heart.

The blood we are now considering has commenced its journey through the body. From the aorta it passes into smaller passages called *Arteries* and is called arterial blood (see Fig. 23). Every time the ventricles contract the blood is pushed farther along. It may go to the head, or stomach, or arms, or legs, or any other part of the body. Farther from the heart, the arteries get smaller and smaller until they become very tiny and are then called *Capillaries*. Here the blood loses its bright red colour owing to loss of oxygen which finds its way through the thin walls of the capillaries into the tissues. Farther along, the capillaries join together again and are now called *Veins*. Like a river with streams feeding it, the veins get bigger and bigger as they get nearer the heart. The blood in them is now impure, having lost much of its oxygen and got in its place CO_2 and waste material from the tissues. It is called venous blood.

Finally, two big veins bring this blood, one from the head and neck and upper parts, and the other from the lower part of the body and legs. The blood in its impure state reaches the heart and enters the *Right Auricle*. This is a thin-walled room and into it comes all the impure blood of the body. When the auricles are squeezed in the heart-beat, the blood in this auricle passes through the door called the *Tricuspid Valve* into the *Right Ventricle*. This room has much thicker walls than the auricle, and when the ventricles are squeezed it forces the blood out, in the same way as the left ventricle did.

The blood cannot pass back again into the auricle as the tricuspid valve only allows it to flow one way; and so the impure dark red blood has to pass out by the *Pulmonary Artery*. This artery goes to the lungs; one branch to the right lung and one to the left. As before, the artery breaks up into capillaries, and, as we saw in the chapter on respiration, the blood in the lung capillaries changes from dark to bright red through taking up oxygen from the air in the lungs. The capillaries lead into veins and finally all of them join to form the *Pulmonary Vein* which carries the pure red blood back to the heart. The pulmonary vein enters the *Left Auricle*, and when the auricles are squeezed during the heart-beat, this pure blood now passes through the mitral valve into the left ventricle, ready to commence its journey round the body once again.

In a grown man the average number of beats to the minute is about seventy, but this is greatly increased in excitement, exercise, fevers or anæmia.

THE BLOOD-VESSELS

We have spoken of Arteries, Capillaries and Veins. The diagram on page 79 will show how they are related one with the other.

The Arteries.—These vessels carry blood away from the heart. They are strong-walled, and will not close up when cut. They are elastic and have some muscle fibres in them; as the heart pumps blood into them they dilate and then contract again. When an artery is cut the blood is seen to be a bright red and it spurts out as the heart beats. (The *Pulmonary Artery* has dark red blood in it but this rarely gets cut as it is deep in the body.) One is in danger of bleeding to death if a large artery is cut, as the walls will not close up by themselves.

Capillaries.—The walls of the capillaries are extremely thin, consisting, in fact, of only one layer of thin cells.

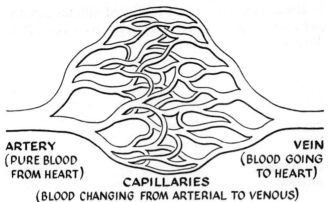

ARTERY
(PURE BLOOD
FROM HEART)

VEIN
(BLOOD GOING
TO HEART)

CAPILLARIES
(BLOOD CHANGING FROM ARTERIAL TO VENOUS)

Fig. 22.—Diagram of Blood-Vessels.

Veins.—These have much thinner walls than the arteries and, if cut, will close up. Hence a cut vein is not so dangerous. Also many of them contain valves which will allow the blood to flow only towards the heart. As they are a long way from the aorta, and the blood before reaching them has had to pass through the narrow capillaries, there is no pulse in the veins, and the blood flows steadily in them.

The blood goes from the left side of the heart to the capillaries and there becomes impure. After this most of it goes straight back to the heart and then to the lungs for purification. The blood, however, which happens to be carried by branches of the aorta to the stomach, intestines and spleen does not follow this course. The capillaries in these organs are, as usual, collected into veins and these unite to form the *Portal Vein*. This, instead of going straight back to the heart, enters the liver, where it breaks up a second time into capillaries. These liver capillaries again unite to form the *Hepatic Vein*, and this vein goes back to the heart.

Hence we see that blood connected with the digestive organs and spleen passes through *two sets* of capillaries before going back to the heart.

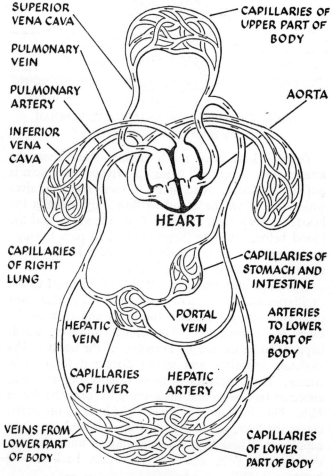

Fig. 23.—Diagram of the Circulation of the Blood.

We must further note that the lungs, besides receiving impure blood for purification, also receive pure blood to give them strength for their work. The liver also, besides receiving impure blood from the digestive system through the *Portal Vein*, receives pure blood by the *Hepatic Artery* to enable it to do its work. The heart has the *Coronary Arteries* to supply its needs.

THE LYMPHATICS

Before closing our study of the blood and its circulation, there is one correction to be made. We said that the blood goes from the capillaries to the veins and then to the heart. But not all the blood does this. In the capillaries some of the plasma escapes into the tissues and nourishes them. The red corpuscles stay in the blood but a few white ones pass out with the plasma. This is now called *Lymph*. It is collected in vessels called *Lymphatics* which are something like veins, and have many valves in them. These lymphatics pass through *glands*. The lymphatic glands can sometimes be felt as lumps in the groin, armpit and neck as they swell up in certain illnesses. This is because the lymphatic vessels and glands produce white corpuscles, whose work is to fight the germs of sickness. Finally the lymphatics join and enter the large veins at the root of the neck. In this way the lymph gets back into the blood.

Chapter 10

THE DIGESTIVE SYSTEM

We now come to another great system of the body—the Food System. This System has been built up to ensure that each organ of the body shall get what food it requires in the form in which it can take it. There are several parts to this system and the organs concerned are the *Mouth, Gullet, Stomach, Small Intestine, Large Intestine* and the *Digestive Glands*.

We shall consider these in turn and see what they do to help. The food we eat cannot be taken into the blood as it is, and the purpose of digestion is to turn our food into such a form that it can enter the blood and be carried by it to the various parts of the body.

We must remember that food contains certain classes of constituents—Proteins, Sugars and Starches, Fats and Oils, Salts, Vitamins and Water (see Chapter 5). Only a portion of, say, a piece of yam is useful to the body. Some of it is indigestible and must be got rid of, and the good part has to be prepared to enter the blood. To understand how this is done needs an outline of the process of digestion.

THE MOUTH

This is where digestion begins. The teeth break up the food so that it may be mixed with saliva and swallowed.

Teeth.—As is well known, we have two sets of teeth.

The first set begin to appear at about seven months of age and are called *Milk Teeth*. Until they come no solid food ought to be given. They are twenty in number. At about six years of age the second set, or permanent teeth, begin to come. These are thirty-two in number. All except four of these will have appeared by about twelve years of age; the last four (*Wisdom Teeth*) are sometimes very late in coming, or may altogether fail to appear.

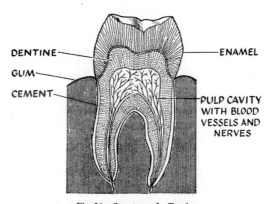

Fig. 24.—Structure of a Tooth.

Structure.—A tooth consists in the main of a hard substance called *Dentine*. Below the gum this is covered by a layer of *Cement*. Above the gum the dentine is covered with a very hard and white substance called *Enamel*. The interior of the tooth is hollow and filled with a soft pulp, in which are small blood vessels and the nerve. When it gets exposed to the air owing to the decay of the tooth the person gets toothache.

Care of the Teeth.—As an aid to digestion as well as to general health it is essential to look after the teeth. *Bad teeth* give great pain while decaying, cause indigestion, and give rise to general ill-health.

The care of the teeth should start with the milk

teeth. It is not right to say " The child is going to lose them anyway, so why look after them? " These teeth have got several years' work to do. If they go bad, the child will not only have pain in them but will not be able to chew his food properly and so will digest it badly. They have another job to do: they have to keep open a spacc in the jaw for the permanent teeth to fit into. If the milk teeth are bad, they decay and disappear too soon, the bone grows differently and there is not enough room for the new teeth to grow properly. The milk teeth should disappear only when the new teeth are forming. The root of the milk tooth slowly gets smaller; its crown stays good until it has no root; then it becomes loose and comes out easily with hardly any pain. It is important, therefore, that children should be trained to look after their teeth.

Three things are known to keep teeth fit: the right food for forming them, hard food for exercising them, and regular cleaning.

1. The diet must be right, and must begin with the mother's diet. When the baby is suckling, and even when it is still in her womb, the mother should have eggs and milk, protein food, such as beans, and ground-nuts and plenty of green food. If she cannot have butter too, remember that red palm oil will provide the necessary vitamins, provided she is in the sun a good deal. By the time a baby is weaned, it should have been eating body-building foods like soup, milk and eggs. Otherwise the enamel may be weak and decay easily.

2. Teeth grow well only if they are used. We must chew our food, and be sure to chew hard things like baked maize or biscuits. Fruit actually helps to clean the teeth as we chew it. Babies start to chew their fingers when their teeth are coming. When this starts,

give them something hard to try to bite, such as a bone; do not let them swallow it.

3. Cleaning is needed, unless our diet is always perfectly arranged. The reason for this being necessary is that germs multiply in little bits of food between the teeth: the germs make an acid which dissolves enamel. They multiply most after the evening meal and before breakfast, because they have the time undisturbed. So we clean our teeth at night, and eat nothing after they are clean. Many people clean them after breakfast as well, and everyone should. But there is no need to clean them before breakfast; they are still clean then if they were cleaned at night.

Chewing sticks and tooth sponges are excellent. Brushes are used for quicker cleaning. They should be used as thoroughly as a chew-stick, however, up and down more than across the teeth. Tooth pastes and powders are pleasant but not very necessary. Some of them do the gums good; some, described as ammoniated, are said to prevent acid from forming.

The Saliva.—This is an alkaline fluid which is poured into the mouth from the *Salivary Glands*, of which there are three pairs situated below the ear, in the cheek and under the tongue. Saliva consists of water, salts, mucus (slime) and the ferment *ptyalin*.

Acids and Alkalies.—We shall have to mention these frequently. An *acid* is a chemical substance which is sharp to the taste. Vinegar is an acid. Acids turn a piece of blue litmus paper a red colour. *Alkalies* are just the opposite of acids. They are soapy to the touch and will turn red litmus blue. Washing soda is an alkali.

G

Ferments.—These are rather mysterious things When sugar is changed into alcohol and carbon dioxide by means of yeast, this is called *fermentation*. When milk goes sour, or meat putrefies, the same kind of thing happens. These changes are produced by germs.

Other kinds of ferment consist of chemical substances. An example of this class is the ptyalin which is produced by the salivary glands. All ferments have the property of changing one substance into another, while they themselves do not change. Ptyalin will only work in an alkaline solution; *Pepsin*, another ferment, needs acid to work in.

Digestion in the Mouth.—Here food is chewed up, mixed with saliva, and made so that it can easily be swallowed. Saliva will not digest proteins or cellulose, but the ptyalin changes starches to sugar. Hence we see the necessity of *chewing our food well*, so that the ptyalin can get at the starch hidden in the starch grains.

THE GULLET OR OESOPHAGUS

From the mouth the food passes into the gullet. This, like the stomach and intestines, is a muscular organ and can force the food along if necessary. A man can drink even when standing on his head. The muscle can reverse its action to produce vomiting. The gullet is about nine inches long and ends in the stomach where the second stage of digestion takes place.

THE STOMACH

The stomach is an elastic bag of the shape shown in Fig. 25. It is lined with what looks like a smooth skin but is seen through the microscope to be full of holes.

These holes do not, of course, go through the stomach wall; they are tube-shaped glands (Fig. 26) and from them is poured *Gastric Juice* when food is to be digested. The stomach increases in size when food goes into it,

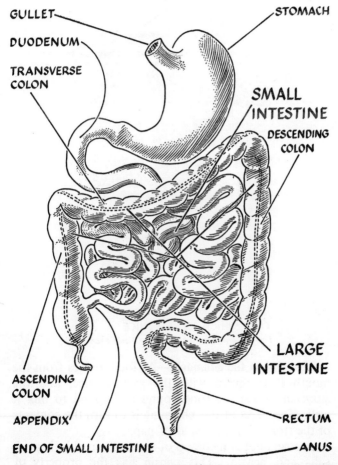

GULLET

DUODENUM

TRANSVERSE COLON

STOMACH

SMALL INTESTINE

DESCENDING COLON

LARGE INTESTINE

ASCENDING COLON

APPENDIX

END OF SMALL INTESTINE

RECTUM

ANUS

Fig. 25.—Stomach and Intestines.

and decreases when empty. Its walls contain fairly strong muscles.

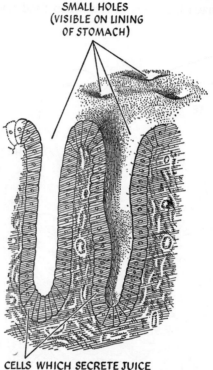

SMALL HOLES
(VISIBLE ON LINING
OF STOMACH)

CELLS WHICH SECRETE JUICE

Fig. 26.—Glands of the Stomach. (Highly magnified.)

Digestion in the Stomach.—As food arrives from the mouth it is mixed with the gastric juice, and the stomach moves the food round and round to mix it well. The effect of this churning is to turn the contents of the stomach into a kind of pap.

Gastric juice is made up of water, hydrochloric acid, salts and pepsin. This pepsin has the property of changing proteins to a form in which they can pass through the stomach wall and be absorbed, going at once to nourish the body.

It also contains a ferment called *rennin* which clots milk, thus preventing it from passing too quickly into the small bowel.

It should be noted that when the food is in the stomach the acid gastric juice " kills " the alkaline saliva, that is, it stops the action of the ptyalin. If a good-sized meal is taken, the gastric juice takes some time to get into the mass of food; so the saliva continues to act for a time. If little bits of food are eaten at odd times, the action of the saliva is stopped at once.

In the stomach, then, starches and proteins are acted on; even they are not digested completely there. The fats and oils are not touched, except that the bags containing the drops of fat and oil are broken and the oil set free. Stomach digestion lasts from one to three hours.

THE SMALL INTESTINE

The food now passes from the stomach into the bowels or intestines. The small intestine is a long tube which when uncoiled measures about 21 feet. It ends by joining the large intestine.

Structure.—The tube of the intestine has an appearance like velvet inside. If looked at through a powerful glass, the " hairs " of the velvet are seen to be as in Fig. 27. Inside are seen blood vessels and a *Lacteal*.

The lacteal leads into a lymphatic vessel, and this, as we have seen in Chapter 9, leads into lymphatic glands and at last into the blood stream. Food passes through the wall of the intestine into the lacteal, and so into the blood. We shall see that this is what happens to the fats and oils.

Two other organs send juices into the small intestine. These juices, the *Bile* and the *Pancreatic Juice*, are produced by the *Liver* and the *Pancreas*.

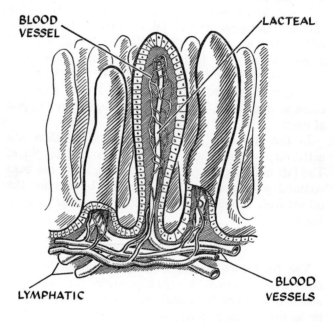

Fig. 27.—Lacteal and Vessels in Intestine.
(Highly magnified.)

The Liver.—This is the largest organ in the body. It weighs three or four pounds. It is situated just underneath the diaphragm rather on the right side. As we have seen, it receives the portal vein bringing blood from the stomach and spleen, and this vein breaks up into capillaries in it. All through the substance of the liver are very fine tubes: these are *Bile Ducts*. Into these the cells of the liver secrete bile, and the bile ducts join together and form the *Common Bile Duct* which carries the bile to the first part of the small intestine,

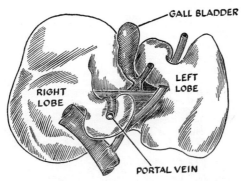

Fig. 28.—The Liver viewed from below, showing Gall Bladder.

called the duodenum. On the way there the duct has a tube leading into it which comes from the *Gall Bladder*. If the bile is not wanted it passes up this tube into the gall bladder and is kept there till required.

Bile.—Bile is a yellow fluid. It contains mucus, water, and special salts called *Bile Salts*. Its work is to act on the fats and oils and to break them up into very small drops so that they look like milk. The bile is also an antiseptic (germ-killer). Bile is sometimes vomited.

Besides producing bile, the liver acts as a storehouse for sugar. When extra sugar is needed by the body for work or violent exercise, or just from fright, the adrenal glands secrete more adrenaline which makes the liver pour sugar into the blood, and so provides extra food for the muscles.

The Pancreas.—This is another large gland; it is called by butchers the sweetbread. It is reddish yellow

in colour and is about seven inches long. It lies behind
the stomach, and a tube from it called the *Pancreatic
Duct* enters the intestine near where the bile duct enters.

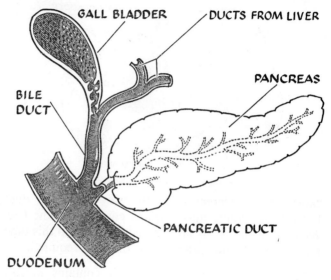

Fig. 29.—Diagram showing Gall Bladder, Pancreas, and Ducts.

Pancreatic juice is a colourless fluid, alkaline, and
containing ferments. These *pancreatic ferments* are
very important. They act on all classes of food—

1. On the Proteins: acting on them just as pepsin
   does.
2. On the Starches: turning them into sugar as
   does ptyalin.
3. On the Fats: turning them into glycerine and
   acids.

We can now see what goes on in the small intestine.
The food is mixed with bile and pancreatic juice,

these juices turn the acid mixture into an alkaline one and stop the pepsin fermentation. Between them they digest proteins, and turn starches into sugar, fats and oils into a milky fluid.

Absorption.—The intestine is not only an organ of digestion, it is also one of absorption. That is, the food, after it has been digested and made so that it can pass through the walls of the intestine, is taken into the blood and then distributed all over the body.

Some passes through the walls of the " hairs " and then is able to enter the little blood-vessels which lie in them, and is carried to the liver. Therefore it gets into the blood quickly.

Fat can pass through the walls of the " hairs " but cannot get through the walls of the blood-vessels. It finds its way into the lacteal in the centre and thence, as explained above, into the lymphatics and blood.

Food remains in the small intestine for about twelve hours. During this time it is being slowly passed on towards the large intestine. This is done by means of a kind of worm-like movement which travels as a wave along the bowel. All this time the digested food is being absorbed.

THE LARGE INTESTINE

This is a tube about 6 feet long. In Fig. 25 you will see that near where the small intestine enters it there is a small blind tube called the *Appendix*. Sometimes this becomes inflamed. This disease is called appendicitis, and can be very serious.

The large bowel is in three parts; the ascending, transverse and descending colons. The end of the bowel is fairly straight and is called the *Rectum* and this ends at the *Anus*, also called the back passage.

Structure.—The large intestine has no " hairs ", but has glands which secrete juice.

Digestion in the Large Intestine.—Food remains in the large bowel from twenty-four to thirty-six hours. There is little digestion done, the main work being the absorption of water and whatever food is left in the material handed on by the small intestine. Through loss of water, the material in the large intestine gets harder as it reaches the rectum and finally the indigestible remnant is turned out, when we open our bowels, as *fæces*, also called *excrement*, or *stools*. The word *excreta* includes stools and urine.

We have now finished looking at the way the food we eat gets into blood in a form which the blood can carry. This food then feeds every part of the body itself. The living cells of the body choose what foods they want and then use them to build themselves up.

Chapter 11

THE EXCRETORY AND CUTANEOUS SYSTEMS

We have now to consider the Excretory System, which is like the Sanitary System of the body. We all know that by emptying our bowels (defæcation) and passing our water (urination) we excrete waste products. But our digestive and our urinary systems are helped by the lungs and the skin.

Importance of this System.—We know that when we make a fire it is necessary now and then to take away the ashes in order that it may burn well. As our bodies do their daily work, " ashes " are formed, and it is necessary that they should be removed. These are the waste products formed by the " burning " of the food carried by the blood to the tissues and have to be got rid of. One of them is Carbon Dioxide, which may be compared with the smoke of the fire.

THE BOWELS

Waste matter which cannot be digested remains in the large intestine in a solid form and is passed as fæces. If the bowels are not open regularly, we say the person suffers from *constipation*; excess of waste matter in the bowel may cause all manner of disease and trouble. Constipation should be guarded against as follows—

1. Take your meals at regular times.
2. Don't over-eat.
3. Take a good amount of exercise.
4. Drink water in the early morning and before you go to bed, but not much at meals. Drink during the day according to need.
5. Eat plenty of fruit and greens.
6. If you feel you want to open your bowels, go and do so at once. Aim to go to latrine regularly at the same time each day.

Occasional constipation may be relieved by taking purgatives, but these should never be taken regularly, for, if a purge-habit is formed, the bowel will refuse to work well unless a purge is given. A person who needs frequent purgatives should consult a doctor, as careful treatment is required, such as a suitable laxative.

THE LUNGS

We have seen that the lungs throw off carbon dioxide and water (as vapour) as well as some organic matter. Thus the lung is an organ of excretion as well as of respiration. It is estimated that over two pounds weight of CO_2 and water is given off daily by the lungs.

THE KIDNEYS

We have not studied these as yet. There are two kidneys, situated one on each side of the back-bone in the small of the back or loin. They are shaped as shown in the sketch and are about four inches long.

The dented part of the kidney is called the *Hilum* and at this place several vessels enter it. There are the renal artery which brings blood, and the renal vein which takes it away; there are the usual nerves and lymphatic vessels, and also a special tube called the *Ureter*. This takes urine from the kidney to the *Bladder*, which acts as a reservoir for urine.

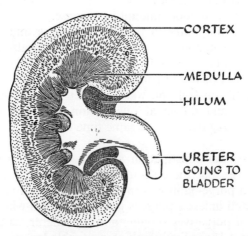

Fig. 30.—Diagram of Kidney and Ureter.

Structure of the Kidney.—The kidney, if opened, is seen to consist of two parts; the outside, or *Cortex*, which is dark in colour, and the *Medulla* (see Fig. 30 on p. 96). The medulla is made up of a vast number of fine tubes leading into the hilum. These tubes are surrounded by capillaries. Their work is to take minute drops of urine from the blood, and pour them into the hilum. From there the urine flows down to the bladder, which gradually fills until we " pass water ".

Urine is normally a pale yellow liquid and is the carrier of the waste nitrogen of the body. We saw that the lungs throw off carbon dioxide and water, and the nitrogen from the inspired air. It is the urine which gets rid of most of the waste nitrogen from our protein foods. Urine also contains mineral salts, chiefly common salt. The quantity of urine passed daily varies according to the temperature, but the amount of waste matter passed does not change much. On hot days the blood flows more to the skin and much water passes off as sweat. But in cold weather more blood goes through the kidneys and so more urine is formed. In hot countries so much water is lost in the form of sweat by the skin that the urine is apt to get too concentrated through lack of water. Hence it is a good thing in a hot country to drink plenty of liquid between meals.

As we have seen, fæces and urine are also called *excreta*.

THE SKIN

We now come to another important organ of the body—the Skin. It has four kinds of work to do—

1. To protect the body.
2. To excrete waste matters.

3. To regulate the temperature of the body.
4. To give us the sense of touch.

Structure.—Skin is composed of two layers.

1. The Outer Layer or Epidermis.—This is the part we see. It protects the inner layer from harm and will not let dirt or water through.

In the palms and soles this layer becomes very thick and horny. We know that we can cut the thick skin of our heels without feeling any pain and without blood flowing. Hence we learn that this layer has no nerves or blood-vessels. The deepest layers of the epidermis contain very small colour grains which in dark-skinned and sunburnt people are dark coloured.

2. The Inner Layer or Dermis.—This layer contains nerves, blood-vessels, hair roots, the organs of touch

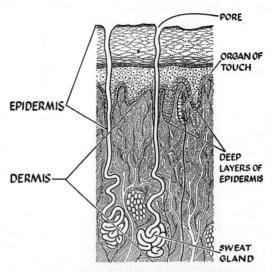

Fig. 31.—Section of the Skin. (Highly magnified.)

and two kinds of gland. Although we are considering the skin now as an organ of excretion, we may as well speak of *the hair* and *sense organs* at this place.

Hairs are outgrowths of the epidermis contained in pits. At the bottom of the pit is the root of the hair and this is connected with the dermis and supplied with blood-vessels. The hair itself consists of horny cells with colour grains in them. This colour is lost in old age and the hair turns white.

The Sense Organs.—These are little lumps in the dermis which are nerve endings. They report to the central nervous system when anything touches, presses upon, heats, cools, pinches or pricks the skin. Where there are a lot of them, the skin is very sensitive.

The Glands of the Skin.—These are of two kinds, the *Sebaceous Glands* and the *Sweat Glands*. The sebaceous glands secrete an oily substance which is

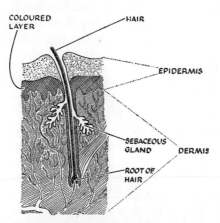

Fig. 32.—A Hair. (Magnified).

poured on to the hair which thinly covers the skin
(Fig. 32). This oil acts as a lubricant and keeps the
skin soft and the hair in good condition. The sweat
glands are the glands which make the skin an organ
of excretion. They are situated all over the skin. Their
openings are the so-called *pores* of the body. The
glands are deep in the dermis and the tube leading
to the surface is coiled up like a corkscrew (see
Fig. 31). Their work is to take up sweat from the blood
and pour it out on the skin. When the sweat reaches
the surface it evaporates and disappears. So long as
there is not a great deal of perspiration all the sweat
is thus got rid of; when, however, we perspire freely,
drops of sweat are seen on the skin.

Composition of Sweat.—Sweat consists mainly of
water. There are also salts (mainly common salt),
fats and bits of skin. The skin and the kidneys thus
work in with one another, as both get rid of much the
same waste products from the body. If more urine
than usual is passed, the skin does less work, and when
there is great perspiration there is less urine. In some
diseases, where the urine is restricted, it is found that
the skin tries to make up for this by excreting more in
the sweat.

CLEANLINESS

Our study of the skin and its functions enables us
to see how important cleanliness is. The surface of
the skin is constantly being fouled not only by dirt
from the outside but also by the secretions of the
sebaceous and sweat glands and bits of the epidermis
that peel off. If these are not cleaned off we get in
time a kind of plaster over the skin consisting of dead

skin, organic matter, dust and grease, which soon becomes smelly and dangerous to health.

Bad effects of uncleanliness.

1. The pores become choked, and the glands put out of action. The other organs of excretion, the lungs and kidneys, have more work thrown upon them.

2. One of the uses of the sweat glands is, as we have seen, to regulate the temperature of the body. The more one sweats the cooler one becomes. But if the glands are put out of action by dirt the heat of the body cannot be regulated properly.

3. Dirt favours the growth of germs and parasites, and these, as we shall see later, give rise to disease.

We shall consider this subject again when we deal with *Personal Health.*

Chapter 12

THE NERVOUS AND OTHER SYSTEMS

THE BONY AND MUSCULAR SYSTEMS

We have not yet said much about how the body moves; this is done by means of *muscles.* The *skeleton* holds the body up and protects those parts of it which could otherwise easily be damaged; it also makes it possible for the body to move properly.

The Skeleton.—We have a very large number of bones. If you start to count the bones in your arm, you find the *shoulder-blade*[1] and *collar-bone*[2] attached to

---

[1] Scapula.   [2] Clavicle.

the *arm-bone*.[1] Then you find two bones in your fore-arm[2], but you cannot count the little bones in your wrist;[3] there are eight of them. Then your hand or palm contains five bones[4] and the fingers and thumb have fourteen.[5]

In the lower half of the body, the *spinal column*[6] is attached below to the *hip-bone*[7] and there are two *thigh-bones*[8] attached to this. Then there is the *knee-cap*.[9] The *shin-bone*[10] has another bone beside it in the leg; this is smaller and is called the *brooch-bone*.[11] There are seven bones in the ankle,[12] five in the instep,[13] and fourteen in the toes.[5]

The *skull* is composed of several bones joined into one; only the *lower jaw* is able to move. The *spinal column* or *back-bone* is made of the spinal bones of the neck,[14] the chest[15] and the loins.[16] Each of the twelve spinal bones of the chest has two *ribs* attached to it. Most of the ribs are attached in front to the *breast-bone*.[17] The collar-bone also meets the breast-bone at the top.

The Muscles.—All the " red meat " in the body either in a man or an animal is the muscle. Muscles are able to contract, and thus bring their ends nearer together. In the body these ends are attached mostly to different bones so that when the muscles contract, the bones have to move. The tongue, womb and heart are muscles.

The big muscle in front of the arm-bone called

---

[1] Humerus.   [2] Ulna and Radius.   [3] Carpal bones.
[4] Metacarpals.   [5] Phalanges.   [6] Vertebral column.
[7] Pelvis.   [8] Femur.   [9] Patella.
[10] Tibia.   [11] Fibula.   [12] Tarsal bones.
[13] Metatarsals.   [14] Cervical vertebrae.
[15] Dorsal or thoracic vertebrae.
[16] Lumbar vertebrae. Below them are the sacrum attached to the pelvis; and the coccyx or tail bones.
[17] Sternum.

the *biceps* pulls the fore-arm upwards and turns the palm upwards too. If you hold a heavy weight in your hand and bend your elbow, you can easily feel your biceps. Every part of the body contains muscles which work in the same way.

THE NERVOUS SYSTEM

This is the most important system of all; it is important because it tells the rest of the body what to do and how to work together.

Where is the nervous system? The digestive system is mostly in one part of the body; the skeleton is easy to find, though we have bones in every limb; but the nervous system is different from these. One part, called the central nervous system, is all in one place— inside the skull and the spine; but the nerves themselves are everywhere in the body. Every part of the body has some. They are there to feel things and tell us what they are like; they tell us about hot and cold things, painful things and so on. The nerves that carry these messages to the brain are called *sensory nerves*. Other nerves are there to carry messages to the muscles and tell them when to work. They are called *motor nerves*. Imagine how quickly those messages have to go if you step on a hot cinder: your foot tells your spinal cord, and a message rushes down to your thigh muscles to move the foot. This is called *reflex action*.

THE CENTRAL NERVOUS SYSTEM

The Brain.—When we feel or hear or see or smell or taste things, it means that a message has reached the brain. Such messages are dealt with by the *cerebrum* (Fig. 33). Usually we want to do something as a result of what we have noticed; to turn our eyes in the direction where we saw something move; to answer what we have heard; to swallow what tastes good, or spit out what tastes bad. These decisions

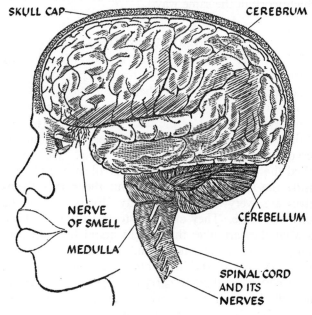

Fig. 33.—The Brain.

and the orders to the muscles are the work of the cerebrum.

The *cerebellum* also looks after the muscles. It makes them work together so that we walk straight and do not fall over when we kick a ball. The third part of the brain is the *medulla*: it sends messages to the heart, lungs and digestive system to keep them working.

Slight damage to the cerebrum may cause blindness or deafness or weakness of muscles. Damage to the cerebellum causes bad balancing. But any damage to the medulla causes death.

The Spinal Cord.—This is like a continuation of the medulla. It runs down the back, surrounded by the bony arch of the spinal column. It consists mostly of nerves which come out of it and run into it between every pair of bones in the spine. But it can also make the simple decisions which are called reflex action.

Special Sense Organs.—Almost any part of our body can *feel*. But our finger cannot tell whether it is light or dark—or whether the baby next door is crying. All the nerves for sight, hearing, taste and smell are kept together in the eyes, ears, tongue and nose—the special sense organs; sight, hearing, taste, smell and feeling are sometimes called the " five senses ".

There are some nerves in your muscles which tell your brain how heavy the things are which they are lifting. This is called *muscle sense*.

The Eyes.—Each of the two nerves for sight spreads itself out in the back of the eye; it forms the *retina* which can tell when light falls upon it. In front of it there is a lens which causes the light which passes through to take the shape of the things in front of us. The lens and the retina are held together and protected by strong and dark coats which make the eye into a ball. These coats have to be transparent in front, where they are called the *cornea*. They are loosely attached to the lids. The eyeball is full of clear water, some of which is so thick as to be more like jelly. It is protected by the *lids* and *eyelashes*. The thing which makes different people's eyes different colours is called the *iris*: this also changes its shape, so as to allow more light to get into the eye in a half-light and to stop too much bright light from getting into the eye. The opening in the middle of the iris is called the *pupil*.

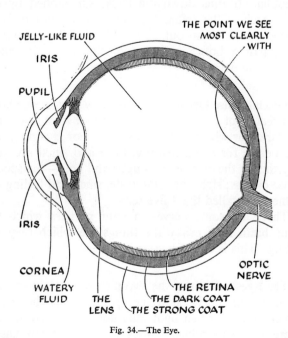

Fig. 34.—The Eye.

The Ears.—The part of our body which hears sounds is a small passage, like a snail-shell, called the *inner ear*. It contains thousands of strings which vibrate when sounds reach them. The *auditory nerve* ends in these strings and tells the brain which ones are vibrating. If you have heard such sounds before, you can tell what is happening. To bring these sounds to the inner ear, the *outer ear* collects them, by means of the *ear-drum*, which passes them through the *middle ear* to the inner ear. There is also a passage from the middle ear to the throat.

With the inner ear is a sense organ for *balancing*. It consists of three *semi-circular canals*. The water in these canals runs about when we move, and the nerve tells the cerebellum which way we have moved. If

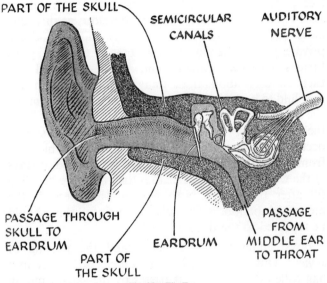

PART OF THE SKULL

SEMICIRCULAR CANALS

AUDITORY NERVE

PASSAGE THROUGH SKULL TO EARDRUM

PART OF THE SKULL

EARDRUM

PASSAGE FROM MIDDLE EAR TO THROAT

Fig. 35.—The Ear.

you turn round several times you get giddy; that is because the water is still running round your semi-circular canals and the nerve is telling the brain that it seems as if you are still moving.

Taste.—The nerves for taste come from the mouth. When anything touches our tongue or palate, these nerves tell the brain whether it is sweet or sour, or bitter or acid.

Smell.—Smells get inside our nose and special nerves send messages to tell the brain what kind of smells they are. Most of these nerves are in the upper part of the nose. That is why we draw air into our nose (sniff) when we want to find what some faint smell is.

THE REPRODUCTIVE SYSTEM

We have already mentioned the main parts of this (see page 3). At the time of *puberty*, that is about 12–14 years, these parts begin to develop; at this time hairs begin to grow in the armpits and around the private parts; the boy's voice breaks and the girl's breasts enlarge. Parents and teachers should tell their children about these things. It is quite right for the child to be curious. Before a girl starts menstruating she should be told what it means. *Menstruation* follows the preparation of the womb for the embryo; it should occur monthly and consist of a few days' bleeding from the birth canal; if the embryo is fertilized, it stays in the womb and grows; there is then no more bleeding till after the child's birth ten months later. If the menstrual period is irregular or painful this should be reported to the doctor.

Boys similarly should understand the passing of *semen*. This is produced in the *testicles* which are in a bag called the *scrotum*. It passes by the same route in the *penis* through which the urine is passed. It begins at adolescence (puberty) and passes at varying intervals throughout life. The function of semen is to *fertilize* the embryo in the mother's womb. Without this contribution from the father, the embryo cannot grow into a baby. Or, as we say, *conception* cannot occur.

What purposes are served by the fact that new life cannot come into being without sexual intercourse of two parents? (1) The baby draws its vitality from two families instead of one. (2) It has two parents instead of one to look after it. A home where husband and wife are devoted to each other and to their children is the starting-place of a full healthy life.

THE SKELETON AND OTHER SYSTEMS 109

further work to do. It has two parts instead
of the single chamber, which we noticed in
the fish. The two parts are the atrium and
[...]

SECTION III

DISEASES

Chapter 13

GERMS

We have learned something of how the body is
organized in its great systems, like the Respiratory,
Circulatory, Digestive and Excretory systems. They
are all organized for the task of carrying on the work
of the body and keeping it in health. We must now
go on to consider the question of ill-health or
disease.

Some diseases such as hare lip are due to faults
in the make-up of our bodies. They cannot be prevented, but once we are aware of them the doctor can
deal with them and perhaps get rid of them altogether.

We are concerned in the study of Hygiene mainly
with diseases which can be prevented, and we must
know something of the causes of these.

PARASITES

One of the chief causes of preventible diseases is the
presence of what are called *Parasites* on or in the body.
The word stands for something which feeds at the
expense of another living thing.

Parasites are familiar to us in the garden or bush.
You often see an orange tree with another tree or
plant living on it. The parasite digs into the trunk of

the tree and drinks some of the sap, and by that means thrives and becomes strong. Sometimes the tree is unharmed, but at other times its strength is taken away and it dies.

But it is not only in the vegetable world that parasites are found. There are also animal parasites. The itch-mite is a parasite, feeding on the bodies of men and animals; so are various worms which live in our bodies. " Ringworm " is not a worm, but a vegetable parasite (see page 165).

GERMS

Germs are a special kind of parasite. They may be animals or plants. The point which interests us most is that they are so small in size that they cannot be seen with the naked eye. We need a powerful microscope to see them at all. Germs are of two kinds, good and bad. Not all of them are troublesome. Some of them live in the intestines and help in the digestion of food; another kind live in the soil and do a great deal to help plants to get their food; others, as we have already seen, help like yeast in fermentation.

It was the French chemist Louis Pasteur who first discovered the part played by germs in nature. He was the first to recognize them under the microscope and to prove their power to cause disease in man. When these get into the body in sufficient numbers they cause disease. In fact all diseases which are infectious, and can pass from one person to another, are caused by germs. Being so hard to see makes them dangerous. Some are too small even to see with the strong microscopes which show us malaria or tuberculosis parasites. They are given the special name of *virus*.

Disease Germs.—These are of different kinds and

each kind produces a special disease. One germ will produce, say, tuberculosis, but will not produce any other disease. The tuberculosis germ can reproduce itself, and its " children " will also be able to cause tuberculosis. Tuberculosis *can only be produced by that kind of germ*. If a person falls sick with that disease we

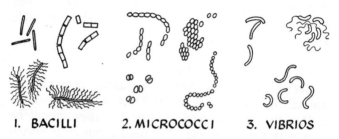

1. BACILLI   2. MICROCOCCI   3. VIBRIOS

Fig. 36.—Classes of Germs. (Very highly magnified.)

know that he has " caught " the germ somehow; the germ has come from some other person, or, more rarely, from an animal.

We see, then, that it is necessary for a *special germ* to be present before the disease it causes can occur. It is not true therefore to say that tuberculosis is due to overcrowding, or that malaria is due to a hot, damp climate. Overcrowding causes people to breathe germs into their bodies. Germs enter in large numbers from a sick person coughing in a crowded room. Similarly, a hot, damp climate favours mosquitoes which carry the malaria parasite.

Groups of Germs.—Germs are of different shapes and are partly classified according to these shapes.

Some of these classes are:

1. Those shaped like small rods called *Bacilli*.

Tuberculosis, typhoid, diphtheria, plague, leprosy and other diseases are caused by germs of this class.

2. Round or oval germs called *Cocci*, or *Micrococci*. The pneumonia germ is of this shape.

3. Germs which are curved in shape called *Vibrios*. The cholera germ is a vibrio.

4. Very small animal parasites are sometimes called germs too: see Malaria, p. 131.

5. Still smaller creatures called *viruses*. Influenza, measles, polio, yellow fever and a number of other diseases are caused by them.

Growth of Germs.—Germs increase very rapidly if they have favourable conditions. They grow by *Division*. One germ divides into two, two into four and so on. At this rate millions of germs can be produced in a few hours.

The following conditions are favourable to the growth of germs:

1. *Warmth.*—Germs require a certain temperature for growth. The temperature of our blood is very suitable for disease germs, for they are fitted for living in our bodies. And most of them live well in the tropics because here the temperature outside the body is often similar to that inside it.

2. *Moisture.*—Germs cannot grow if they are dry. Dampness is favourable to them. In the wet season one's boots become coated with mould which is really a collection of millions of harmless parasites. In the dry season this does not occur.

3. *Food.*—Like other living creatures they need food. When they are outside the body, the most common food of germs is decaying animal or vegetable matter. That is one reason why dirty water, sewage or bits of food must not be left about.

HOW TO KILL GERMS

We can kill germs, or render them harmless, by taking away the above conditions.

1. Heat.—No germs can live long in the temperature of boiling water. Boiling an infected article makes it *sterile*, that is, free from living parasites. Most germs cannot fight very well at fever temperature; that is why the body has a fever when germs are trying to attack it, and why fomentations help.

2. Cold.—We know that ice prevents food from fermenting. Germs can be stopped from increasing by cold; but we cannot be sure they are killed.

3. Sunlight.—Most germs cannot stand sunlight, while all love darkness. Hence the importance of allowing plenty of sunlight to enter our rooms. On the other hand there are germs, like that of diphtheria, which do not mind sunlight.

4. Cleanliness.—A great many germs feed on filth, such as germs of typhoid, cholera, diphtheria and blood poisoning. The germs of lockjaw live in horse manure, and soil. So cleanliness is their great enemy.

5. Fresh Air.—Oxygen is an enemy to most germs.

6. Antiseptics or Disinfectants.—These substances kill germs by poisoning them. They are very important.

It was the Scottish surgeon Lister who first found out how to use them in surgery so as to prevent germs infecting the wounds. Although surgeons no longer use a carbolic spray over the wound as he did, we use similar antiseptics to kill germs.

Lysol is used mixed with water in varying strengths. The strongest is one in forty.[1] It is a good antiseptic in this form. Of course the smell will not kill a germ, it must be the liquid itself.

Dettol is another popular disinfectant. A teaspoonful to a pint of water is useful for cleaning.

Some chemicals are very useful in that while they are hardly strong enough to kill powerful germs they will not allow germs to grow where they are. They are not irritating to the flesh and can be used for washing out dirty wounds, which soon heal under their influence. Among these are *Tincture of Iodine*, solutions of potassium permanganate or cetrimide in water; *Boric Acid*, a white medicine which is either used as a powder or as crystals dissolved in water (Boracic Crystals dissolve better than the powder); and *Iodoform*, a yellow substance which is much stronger and is used as a powder. Iodoform should never be used by itself. Mixed with 5 or 10 times as much boric acid powder it is an excellent antiseptic for bad ulcers. Others such as *Acriflavine* and *Aureomycin* are also used for wounds and are very effective.

Thus we see that there are many ways of killing germs before they get into the body. But we ought not to rely on antiseptics to keep us free from germs. The best method is that which can be used by everyone at little cost, namely the *method of cleanliness*. Plenty of *fresh air*, *sunlight*, and *soap and water* will make it almost impossible for certain germs to grow, and these means are our best preventives against disease.

But doctors led by Sir Alexander Fleming, the discoverer of *Penicillin*, have now found many drugs called *Antibiotics* which will kill off germs after they have got into our bodies, when taken by mouth or injection.

[1] Two teaspoons to a pint.

HOW GERMS ENTER THE BODY

We all know that we catch some diseases from other people. This is not because we believe in "the evil eye" or witchcraft, but because germs from a sick person can get out of him into a healthy person. Diseases which can be caught in this way are called *Communicable Diseases* because they can be communicated or passed on. Some diseases can also be caught from animals or birds.

If germs succeed in getting in and living and breeding in us we become *infected*, and then we in our turn may become *infectious* to others. There are four main ways in which germs can enter the body and we can class diseases accordingly:

1. Air-borne Diseases.—These are carried by germs in the small droplets in the breath. So we may breathe them in direct from the sick person if we get close to him, or we may inhale them in the dried-up dust of infected spit which may get blown about the room or the streets. The common cold and most of the infectious diseases of children, the so-called school diseases, and also *Tuberculosis*, are air-borne diseases.

2. Insect-borne Diseases are carried by two-winged biting flies or by mosquitoes, or other insects such as fleas, lice, ticks and mites. The germs are not just carried by insect hosts, but live part of their lives in them and breed in them. Malaria, Yellow Fever, Sleeping Sickness and Filaria are all insect-borne.

3. Food and Water-borne Diseases are caught by swallowing germs which have got into our drinking water, milk or other foods, either from the excreta of sick people or from those who may have recovered but are still " carriers " of the germs. Also from food exposed to house flies. The dysenteries and typhoid fevers are examples of water-borne diseases.

4. Contact Diseases or Contagious Diseases are carried by germs from sores, or in pus getting smeared into the skin especially if there are uncovered scratches or wounds. Yaws, ringworms and septic sores are common examples. *Venereal Diseases* are generally caught by sexual contact between men and women. House flies can drop germs in our eyes or in wounds.

ACTION OF DISEASE GERMS IN THE BODY

Once the disease germs get inside the body they begin to develop. It is some time before the disease appears and this time, varying with different germs from four to about twenty-one days, is called the *incubation period*. During this period the germs are rapidly increasing in number. The patient feels well and there are no signs of sickness. The germs are producing poisons; each special germ produces its own kind of poison, and it is this poison which produces the symptoms of the disease.

The body, however, is not idle. Some of the white corpuscles attack the germs as was explained when we studied the blood (page 74). If the corpuscles are healthy, and the germs are not too numerous or strong, it is possible that the germs will be eaten up and the disease not be developed. On the other hand if those corpuscles which fight the germs are defeated, the disease commences. The patient is full of germs and is a centre of infection. He may throw off germs in his breath; or in his fæces and urine, which must be disinfected by mixing with some disinfectant. Sometimes the germs keep mainly to the blood (as in malaria) and they can

I

only infect other people by first going into the stomach of an insect (in this case a mosquito), which bites the patient, and then later bites another person.

But even if defeated in the first fight, the body still struggles against the germs. The cells of the tissues and the corpuscles produce a substance that acts as a poison to the germs. Such substances are sometimes called antibodies. If the body is strong enough to produce enough of this the germs are defeated and the patient gets better. If insufficient antibody is produced the patient dies.

Immunity.—We know that if a person has had smallpox once he rarely gets it again. The same thing happens with some other diseases. Why is this? It must be because there are things in his body which kill the germs of that disease as soon as they enter. It is natural to suppose that these things are the medicines which were produced in his body during the first attack of the disease, and which have been kept in store in case of a second attack. We say that the man is *immune*. Immunity for the future may thus be a result of the disease itself. It is comforting for a person who has had smallpox, typhoid or measles to know that he is unlikely to get it again even if it attacks his town.

Inoculation.—There is, however, a better way of acquiring immunity than by suffering from an attack of the disease. It is really somewhat similar, but in this case we introduce the germ into our bodies purposely. We are careful however to see that the germ we introduce will do us no harm. In the case of smallpox the germ used is a feeble one from the body of a calf. In the case of typhoid *dead germs* are introduced, and it is found that although the germs are dead the body will still produce the correct medicine and thus render the man immune. Sometimes instead of putting germs into the person the antibody itself is put in. This is got from the serum of animals which have had the germs put into them, thus saving the man's body the trouble of producing its own. People can be rendered immune to quite a number of diseases by the use of a *vaccine* (as the feeble germs are called) or *serum* (as the other kind is called). Unfortunately, the time for which the person is immune is not lifelong. It lasts about seven years for smallpox, two years for typhoid and shorter times than these for other diseases.

Other Vaccines.—Vaccines are now prepared against Plague, Cholera, Yellow Fever, Diphtheria, Whooping Cough, Tetanus, Polio and Tuberculosis, and these should be used when advised by doctors.

Summary: Prevention of Disease.—Our study of parasites and germs has shown us that we can get rid of a great deal of disease if we prevent germs from reaching our bodies. We have seen that they can enter the blood by the skin, the mouth, the nose and the urinary passages. We must see that they do not get the chance to do so. Our study of water showed us how to obtain clean water so that we should be safe from such germs as those of cholera and typhoid. While studying air we saw that fresh air and good ventilation help to protect us from tuberculosis and other diseases spread by air-carried germs. There are other ways in which germs are carried and these have also been mentioned: (*a*) by insects; (*b*) by dirt. We have now to study in more detail how we can save ourselves from infection by these things.

Chapter 14

AIR-BORNE DISEASES

" Coughs and sneezes spread diseases." This is very true of air-borne diseases, especially among school-children. When someone has one of these diseases he is spreading germs about. Anyone who has been close to him, even on the day or two before the disease has shown itself, has quite likely caught the germs and he may go down with it at the end of the *incubation period* which is the time taken by germs to grow in the body before you get sick. If you know how long this period is you will know when to look for the early signs of the disease in him. Until it has passed we speak about him being in *quarantine* which is counted from the earliest date of contact to the last day of the incubation period. The germs are scattered about by the patient for some days or weeks and this time is called the *isolation period* during which he is infectious to others, even though he may be feeling better. Most of these infectious diseases can only be caught once, because we have become immune.

The Common Cold is easily caught and causes the nose to run and then get blocked up by swelling inside and a thick discharge. It may go down " on to the chest " causing coughing and fever. Unfortunately it gives little or no immunity.

Influenza or the " Flu " is also very infectious. It causes fever and headache and sometimes a bad cough (pneumonia) and stomach upsets.

Sore Throat may spread among crowded classes and cause pain on swallowing. The germs may also damage the kidneys, or cause pain and abscess in the ear.

There are no very good vaccines against colds, influenza or sore throats, though medicines can help to prevent complications.

Diphtheria is a bad disease caused by a germ which can grow in and block the air passages in the throat and choke people. It used to be a common cause of death among children before we had the proper vaccine for it. Incubation period is 2 to 10 days.

Whooping Cough makes a child cough and cough and cough till he loses his breath and at last breathes in with a whooping sound. It may also make him vomit after the bout of coughing so that he gets thin. It may also damage the lungs and cause a weak chest. There is a good vaccine which is usually given mixed with that for diphtheria. Incubation period is 6 to 18 days. Isolation lasts until the cough has practically gone.

Mumps is very catching and generally shows first by bad swelling below the ear, spreading to the salivary gland beneath the jaws. Later it may cause swelling of the testicle or the ovary. The incubation period is long, 21 days, and the isolation period lasts two weeks.

Measles starts with a running nose and eyes, fever and cough. After four days spots or blotches appear on the face, body and limbs. The cough may turn to pneumonia and be fatal if not treated properly. Measles often leads to malnutrition or Kwashiorkor. Incubation period 7 to 14 days. Isolation 7 days.

Rubella (German Measles) is milder and causes swelling of the lymph glands behind the ear and later a measly rash. It does not harm children much, but if a woman who has just got pregnant gets it, her baby may be born with some defect. Incubation 5 to 21 days.

Chicken-Pox is generally a mild disease showing itself by little blebs appearing on the chest and back on the first day, with mild fever. As the spots can resemble those of smallpox, a doctor should decide what it is if possible. Incubation is 11 to 21 days, and isolation lasts till the scabs are off.

Smallpox has been known all over the world as a deadly infectious disease since the dawn of history. It starts with fever and headache and pain in the back, then come blebs or pocks which show first on the face and hands or arms and spread to cover most of the body. Later the blebs get full of pus—pustules, and the fever gets worse and is often fatal. It was the famous Dr. Jenner in England who, having learned that the girls employed in milking cows on the farms did not catch smallpox, explained this by the fact that they had previously caught the cowpox, a similar but mild disease of cattle, which was also called vaccinia. He later proved that by vaccinating healthy people with the germ of vaccinia of cows he could prevent them catching smallpox. Smallpox vaccination lasts about 7 years, but travellers have to be re-vaccinated every three years to make sure that they do not catch the disease again. Smallpox is so infectious that it can be caught from the dead body of a victim or from his clothing, bedding or scabs. Moreover there is no known medicine which will prevent people dying of it, though some do recover from mild attacks. The incubation period is 10 to 14 days, usually 12, and isolation lasts till all scabs fall off. As vaccination "takes" in seven days, those

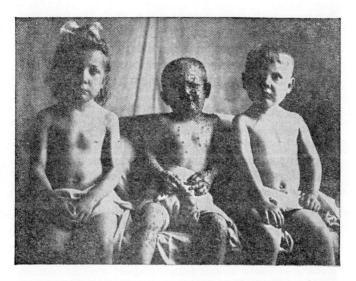

Fig. 37.—From a photograph of three members of a family brought to an Isolation Hospital with their mother who was suffering from smallpox. The child in the centre was *unvaccinated*, the other two had been vaccinated the year before. The two vaccinated children remained in the smallpox wards several weeks and never contracted the disease.

who have come into contact with a case of smallpox can be protected if they are vaccinated without delay.

Meningitis or spotted fever is a disease which can also be fatal. Starting with a headache and a stiff neck it soon causes people to become unconscious. Fortunately the sulphonamide tablets often made available by the Government in rural districts can cure this disease and prevent contacts from catching it. Incubation 5 days, isolation 7 days.

Poliomyelitis (Infantile paralysis).—The germs of this disease are common among people who live in lands without modern sanitation. Children early get some immunity to it and may not suffer, while the foreigner may get bad attacks and lose the use of limbs or die. It is difficult to recognize the disease till weakness of muscles comes on. Incubation is commonly from 7 to 14 days. Fortunately there are now good vaccines.

Tuberculosis, commonly called TB, is the most serious and widespread air-borne disease in the world today. It was in 1880 that the German scientist Dr. Koch discovered the little rod-shaped germ often called *Koch's bacillus*. These germs often affect the lungs and cause a chronic cough with spitting of phlegm and blood. Patients get feverish and thin and weak and often die of it. The germs may cause swelling of the glands in the neck, or may get into the bones of the spine causing deformity. Fortunately we now have good medicines to cure tuberculosis and X-rays to discover it in the lungs and also a vaccine B.C.G. to prevent it. The more advanced countries are quickly getting rid of TB. Bad cases have to be treated in special hospitals, but mild cases can be treated in their own homes or as out patients.

Chapter 15

THE MOSQUITO AND MALARIA

The mosquito is well known and has always been regarded as an enemy because of its bite, which often produces a painful swelling. But we now know that the mosquito is to be feared not so much for the pain of its bite as for the diseases which sometimes follow it.

There are two main varieties of mosquito, and it

has been proved by medical men that certain kinds of these are able to carry the germs of certain diseases and, by their bite, are able to transfer the germ to human beings and animals. For example—

Anopheles mosquitoes carry Malaria.
Culex   „   „   Filaria, Dengue and
                                   Yellow Fever.

Mosquitoes are not the only insects which carry disease germs. Several diseases are caused by flies of

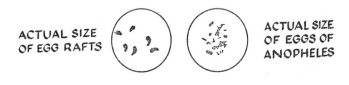

ACTUAL SIZE OF EGG RAFTS

ACTUAL SIZE OF EGGS OF ANOPHELES

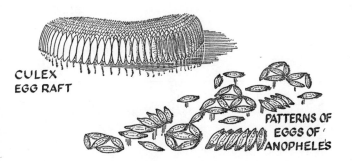

CULEX EGG RAFT

PATTERNS OF EGGS OF ANOPHELES

Fig. 38.—Mosquito Eggs.

different sorts: the *tsetse fly* spreads sleeping sickness; the *tick* carries relapsing fever; *lice* carry typhus; *rat fleas* carry plague; and the common *house-fly* may infect food with germs of typhoid, dysentery and cholera.

THE LIFE-HISTORY OF A MOSQUITO

A man is born as a baby and the baby has the same form as the man. But this is not the case with a mosquito; it has not always had wings and the shape we know so well. The mosquito has four stages of life—the egg, the *larva*, the *pupa* or *cocoon* and the *mosquito*.

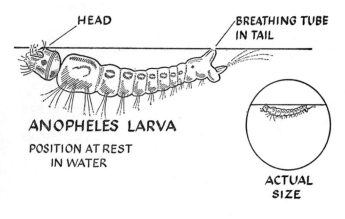

HEAD

BREATHING TUBE
IN TAIL

ANOPHELES LARVA

POSITION AT REST
IN WATER

ACTUAL
SIZE

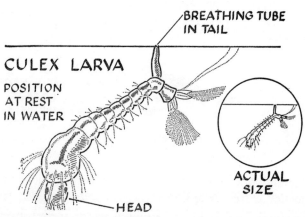

BREATHING TUBE
IN TAIL

CULEX LARVA

POSITION
AT REST
IN WATER

ACTUAL
SIZE

HEAD

Fig. 39.—Mosquito Larvæ.

1. The Egg.—The mosquito lays its eggs on the surface of water. The eggs of the Culex are *oval* and are bunched together in hundreds. The eggs of the Anopheles are *boat-shaped* and are found singly on the water, or in geometrical patterns.

2. The Larva.—In about three days the egg opens and the larva comes out. The larva is of the shape shown in Fig. 39. It consists of a head and a long ringed body. The larvæ of the Anopheles and Culex can easily be distinguished. The Anopheles larva lies at the surface of the water, its whole body quite

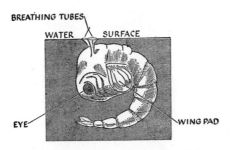

Fig. 40.—Mosquito Pupa. (Ten times natural size.)

flat and touching the surface. The Culex on the other hand dips its head and body beneath the surface in a slanting direction, only its " tail " touching the surface. The " tail " of the Anopheles is shorter than that of the Culex. These " tails " are really breathing tubes which have to pierce the surface when air is required. The larvæ do not always stop at the surface of the water. They wriggle about in search of food. They need a lot of food and are continually eating rotted water plants, insects and so on. The larva grows and sheds its skin now and then until it is full-grown.

The Pupa or Cocoon.—The change from egg to pupa takes about 7–10 days. The larva sheds its skin when full-grown and the perfect pupa comes out. It is hard to distinguish the pupa of the Anopheles from that of the Culex. They are both shaped like a comma,

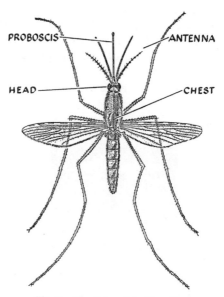

Fig. 41.—Female Anopheles Mosquito.

and from the " head " of the comma come out two short breathing tubes which go to the surface for air. The pupa, like the larva, is a wriggler; but, as it does not feed at all, it stays at the surface unless disturbed.

After a few days the skin of the pupa splits and the perfect mosquito comes out. It rests on the empty skin which acts as a kind of raft, spreads its wings and flies away.

The Structure of the Mosquito.—There are very many kinds of mosquitoes but they all have much the same appearance. The following is a general description of them. We will consider the distinguishing marks of the Anopheles and Culex afterwards.

The Head.—From the female's head projects a straight sharp *proboscis*; also the *feelers*, or *antennae*, and between them some guides for the proboscis.

The Chest carries the muscles which move the legs and wings. There are six legs under the chest and two wings above it.

The back part of the mosquito is made up of rings (usually nine) and contains the organs of digestion and of reproduction.

To distinguish Male and Female.

1. The feelers of the male are more feathery than those of the female.

2. The female has its proboscis longer than its feelers; whereas the proboscis of the male is shorter.

To distinguish Anopheles and Culex.

Size.—*Anopheles* is usually smaller than *Culex*.

Wings.—The wings of the *Culex* are clear. Those of the *Anopheles* are spotted in many cases.

Humming.—The *Anopheles* darts about quickly and almost noiselessly. It does not hum like the *Culex*.

Position.—When at rest on a wall the *Anopheles* has its proboscis and body in a straight line and appears to be digging its head into the wall. The *Culex* has its body parallel with the wall, and its proboscis is not straight with the body. This gives it a hunch-backed appearance.

Habits of Mosquitoes.

1. It will be understood from what we have learned of the life of a mosquito that water is necessary for them. The kind of water most of them choose for laying their eggs in is still water—just the kind which is found at the edges of creeks and lagoons, in old tins and other things often found in an untidy compound.

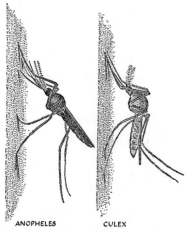

ANOPHELES CULEX

Fig. 42.—Anopheles and Culex at Rest. (Magnified.)

Some *Anopheles* can breed in running water. Some "wrigglers", if thrown on to damp earth, keep alive and develop into mosquitoes when it rains again.

2. Mosquitoes like the juice of plants. The female, however, is fond of blood and will drink that of men or animals in preference to anything else, especially when she has eggs developing in her body. The male does not bite; he is a vegetable feeder. For this reason, malaria can only be passed on by the female.

3. With the exception of one kind of Culex, mosquitoes are not active during the daytime. This kind

is called *Aëdes* (formerly Stegomyia). The majority rest during the day and come out to feed at sundown. In dark rooms, however, they are active during the day also.

4. When a mosquito bites a person he feels it. This is due not to the bite itself but to saliva which the mosquito injects into the wound. It prevents the blood near the bite from clotting, so that the mosquito can drink it.

MALARIA

We have now considered the mosquito and its habits. The insect is interesting to us mainly because it carries the germ which causes malaria. This fever is one of the most widespread of diseases and causes a great deal of sickness and death. Even when it does not prove fatal it may so weaken a person that he is liable to catch other diseases. Children especially are hurt by this disease. They do not possess great powers of resistance, and easily get fever.

Malaria is found practically everywhere, and is said to cause the death of millions of people yearly. Though found chiefly in hot climates it is not confined to them. At one time it was common in England, where it was called ague. There are still occasional cases of it in parts of England where Anopheles mosquitoes are found.

The Cause of Malaria.—Until 1880, no progress was made towards finding the cause of this disease. In that year a French army doctor named Laveran discovered that if the blood of a man suffering from fever was examined under a powerful microscope, small parasites could be seen. Other doctors then did the same and it was found that these parasites were always to be seen in the blood of a malaria patient. How did the parasite get into the blood?

In 1894 Sir Patrick Manson, after studying the behaviour of the parasite in the blood, suggested that it must have been living in the body of some other creature before entering the man. Sir Patrick said the other creature was a mosquito, and that the parasite got into the man from the mosquito. This idea was at first laughed at, as many new ideas are.

Another doctor, Sir Ronald Ross, undertook to prove the ideas of Sir Patrick. He obtained some birds suffering from a fever similar to human malaria and allowed mosquitoes to bite them. He then examined the bodies of the mosquitoes under a microscope and found that some malaria parasites from the birds were living in their stomach walls.

He watched these parasites very carefully and discovered that they changed in a remarkable way and at last found their way into the salivary glands of the mosquito. From these glands the parasites could pass into the proboscis and from it into another bird bitten by the mosquito. The bird would then get the disease and the parasite would be found in its blood. Sir Ronald found that the time taken for the parasite to change from its form when first entering the mosquito to its form when it was ready to infect other birds was about eight days.

These experiments were very important and it only remained to prove that what happened in the case of men was the same as happens in birds. This was proved by some Italian doctors and confirmed by Sir Patrick, who first thought of the mosquito as the carrier.

This is how he proved it:

(1) Some Anopheles mosquitoes which had bitten a

malaria patient in Italy were brought to England. Two Englishmen who had never been to a malarial country allowed themselves to be bitten by these mosquitoes. The men were Dr. Thorburn Manson (son of Sir Patrick) and Mr. R. Warren of the London School of Tropical Medicine. After eighteen days both men were attacked by malaria and the parasites of the disease were found in their blood. This experiment proved that the Anopheles mosquito can carry the germ of malaria, and by its bite give the disease to men.

(2) A party of Sir Patrick's friends went and lived in a place where nearly everyone had malaria. There, during the months when malaria was commonest, they worked hard side by side with people who had the disease; they drank the same water and ate the same food as these people, and took no quinine. *But* they stayed in a big mosquito net from sundown to sunrise, and were not bitten by mosquitoes. None of them caught malaria. This was to prove that malaria is only caught if mosquitoes are allowed to bite people, and not from bad air, bad food, bad water, overwork or the hot sun.

The Life of the Malaria Parasite.—This is a very small animal and it has a very interesting life history.

Let us trace the life of one of these parasites from the time it is introduced into the human body by the bite of an infected female Anopheles mosquito.

1. Life in Man.—The parasites which get into the blood travel around until they fasten on to a suitable cell. When they stop in the liver, they grow very fast and divide into a very large number of parasites rather like themselves. During this time the person who was bitten has no fever. Then this large number of parasites

K

are set free in the blood. Each parasite attacks a red blood corpuscle which it enters. It eats up part of the blood corpuscle and grows. The parasite soon breaks up into little balls called *spores*, which arrange themselves in the form of a rosette. The wall of the blood

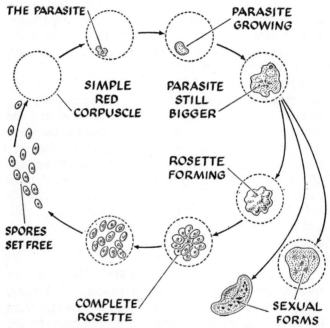

THE PARASITE

PARASITE GROWING

SIMPLE RED CORPUSCLE

PARASITE STILL BIGGER

ROSETTE FORMING

SPORES SET FREE

COMPLETE ROSETTE

SEXUAL FORMS

Fig. 43.—Life of the Malaria Parasite in the Blood. (Highly magnified.)

corpuscle breaks and the spores and poison formed in the corpuscle all escape into the plasma.

It is just after the spores burst that the patient's temperature rises. He feels cold; he shivers and his teeth may chatter. But his forehead is dry and hot. Then he begins to feel warm; he perspires, and feels a lot better. All this takes a few hours, and is called a *rigor*. During this time, the spores try to enter new red corpuscles, but many of them are eaten up by the white blood corpuscles. Some, however, succeed in getting into the red cells and the same thing takes place as before.

The time taken for a parasite to change from the rosette form to another rosette in another red corpuscle is either two or three days, according to the variety of malaria parasite. The spores multiply and destroy red cells; the patient soon suffers from a lack of these cells. He gets pale and anæmic and liable to catch other diseases.

But this is not the end of the history of the parasite. Some of the parasites in the red corpuscles, instead of forming rosettes, turn into so-called *sexual forms*. This is the form which, when it enters the stomach of a mosquito, makes it dangerous to man.

2. Life in the Mosquito.—Let us follow this form of the parasite as it travels with the blood which the mosquito sucks up through its proboscis. Some of these parasites are male and some female. When they get into the mosquito's stomach they soon begin to change their shapes. They become more like balls. Then the male forms throw out from themselves a number of whip-like, wriggling streamers, and the female forms settle on the mosquito's stomach wall.

After a time the male streamers break off and each wriggles about until it meets one of the female or egg cells. This it enters, and so fertilizes the egg. Soon an enormous number of little needle-like bodies develop in this egg. These are also called *spores*. After a time the egg bursts and the spores are set free in the body of the mosquito. They travel about its body and some enter the *salivary glands* which are situated in the mosquito's chest. When the mosquito bites anyone some of these spores are injected with the saliva into the bite and thus enter the human body.

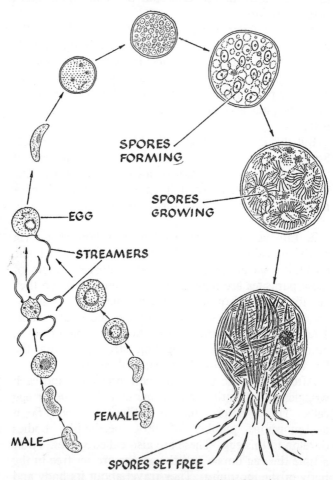

SPORES
FORMING

SPORES
GROWING

EGG

STREAMERS

FEMALE

MALE

SPORES SET FREE

Fig. 44.—The life of the Malaria Parasite in the Mosquito.

The time taken for the sexual forms from a malaria patient to change into spores inside the mosquito is about eight days.

We have now completed the story of the parasite's life. We see it consists of two stages. (1) The stage in the body of a man. (2) The sexual stage in the body of a mosquito.

THE PREVENTION OF MALARIA

As we now know something of the mosquito and of the malaria parasite, we are able to make plans whereby the spread of the disease can be prevented. We shall consider this under several headings:

1. DESTRUCTION OF MOSQUITOES

In some countries, nowadays, all the Anopheles, or all the specially dangerous ones, are prevented from breeding. Usually, all we can do is to reduce their numbers in districts where people are living. Let us first see how we can fight the mosquito. We know the female requires standing water where she may lay her eggs, and where the larvæ and pupæ may grow. The following methods will help:

1. No Standing Water.—Water should not be allowed to stand near our houses. The usual places where water collects are old tins, broken pots and bottles, coconut shells, stumps of banana trees, gutters of corrugated iron roofs and so on. Puddles of water after rain should be drained or filled up with earth. The latrine especially should be kept clean and dry. The kitchen is a place of special danger as people are inclined to throw waste water around it, making the ground sodden. All jars and refuse should be cleared away daily.

2. Drained Surroundings.—The land around our village or town should be free from standing water. Often this means a good deal of work. Where there are large holes formed by digging mud for buildings, an effort must be made to fill them in with rubbish. If the land is swampy it can often be drained by cutting channels through the swamp and letting the water run in them. Places which have been quite uninhabitable owing to mosquitoes and malaria have been made healthy by these simple means.

3. Use of Oil.—Sometimes it is impossible to fill in or drain the land. In this case we have another method of attack. Oil is sprayed on the water. It remains floating and spreads over the whole surface. We have seen that both the larva and pupa of the mosquito have to breathe air by their breathing tubes. If there is oil on the water they cannot breathe, so they suffocate and die. As it takes over a week for the egg to turn into a mosquito, it is sufficient if the pools are oiled once a week.

4. Clearing the Bush.—Besides attacking the larvæ and pupæ we can do much to banish the mosquito itself by clearing away all long grass near the house or village. This destroys the shade in which the mosquito rests.

5. Attack the Mosquito.—When female mosquitoes are getting ready to lay their eggs they must have a blood meal, so they enter our homes and try to feed on us when it is dark. If the inside walls of our houses are sprayed with an *insecticide* like D.D.T., gammexane, dieldrin or chlordane, the mosquitoes will be poisoned when they rest on them. The poison gets in through their feet and then up to their heads so that they die after a few hours. One spraying lasts for many months, but some mosquitoes seem to get used to one insecticide so that it is sometimes necessary to use a different spray.

2. THE MOSQUITO NET

This is one of the chief ways in which we can prevent the spread of malaria. It acts in two ways—(a) by preventing the mosquito from infecting a man by its bite, and (b) by preventing the mosquito from taking the sexual form of the parasite from a malaria patient.

How to use a Net.
  (1) The net should be tucked under the mattress or mat.
  (2) It should have its edges of calico, so that the mosquito is less likely to bite the sleeper's arms or legs if they touch the net.
  (3) It should be put down before dark so that mosquitoes may not get inside as it is being arranged.
  (4) It should be inspected before being slept in and any stray insects inside it killed.
  (5) All holes should be mended. Patching with netting is better than tying up the holes.
  (6) Babies should be inside the net from sunset to sunrise.

Even if we do not generally use a net we ought certainly to use one when suffering from fever. If we do not we may infect some mosquitoes, and these may later on infect someone else.

To prevent being bitten before we go to bed, a good plan is to screen with mosquito wire a part of the house, say a part of the verandah, where we may sit after dark without fear of being bitten. Better still, of course, have the whole house mosquito-proofed. Mosquito wire made of copper is much better than that made of iron, which does not last long.

3. THE USE OF PREVENTIVE MEDICINE

Where malaria is common, it is wise to take medicine against it; but only use this method if you can keep it up regularly.

PREVENTIVE MEDICINES AGAINST MALARIA

Name	Other names	Average adult dose
Chloroquine	Nivaquine, aralen, camoquin, avlochlor	2 tablets once a week
Daraprim	Pyrimethamine	1 tablet once a week
Daraclor	Mixture of above	1 tablet once a week
Paludrine	Proguanil	1 tablet daily
Mepacrine	Atebrin	1 tablet daily
Quinine		1 tablet daily

Daraclor is probably the best of these.

Children up to three years should be given a quarter of the adult dose, and children from four to twelve half the adult dose.

TREATMENT OF MALARIA

People who are taking regular preventive drugs may never get fever. Sometimes, however, if heavily bitten or in poor health the parasites may be able to grow in their blood and cause mild fever. By taking an extra dose or two of the drug they will soon get better, though this is less true of Daraprim. On the whole it is better to follow a stated course of treatment.

Those who live in an area where malaria abounds and have had attacks on and off since childhood are fairly immune against their own type of fever and all they may need is a tablet or two to put them right.

Others who are only partly immune from rare attacks in the past need a little more. But non-immune folk, whether white or black or brown, who have never had malaria before are apt to suffer from severe attacks if they are infected without having been taking a preventive drug. They need urgent treatment with three tablets of chloroquine a day for three days.

It must not be forgotten that preventive drugs only protect as long as they are being taken. If school children stop taking them when they go home on their holidays, they may get dangerous fevers.

Chapter 16

OTHER INSECT-BORNE DISEASES

1. FILARIA

Some blood-sucking insects such as mosquitoes, midges and larger cattle flies can by biting us infect us with minute embryos which may then grow up inside us into adult male and female filarial worms. These may live in our lymphatic glands or other tissues and breed myriads of minute larvae, called microfilariae because they are so small. These swarm in the blood or lymph vessels under the skin where they can be picked up again by the bite of the same kind of insect which gave us the parent worms. After a period of growth and change in the insect's stomach they wriggle to near its mouth and so are able to infect someone else who may be bitten, thus completing the man–fly cycle of reproduction. There are many varieties of filaria, but there are three important and troublesome ones.

1. Filaria causing elephantiasis (*Bancrofti*).—It was Sir Patrick Manson who in 1878 discovered that a mosquito of the culex type carried this filaria. The

embryos wriggle up from the place bitten and get
caught in the nearest lymphatic gland where they grow
up into small worms about two or three inches long.
This causes a blocking of the lymph flow through the
gland so that the area drained gets all " waterlogged "
and swollen and looks like elephant's skin, hence the
name elephantiasis. Their numerous offspring or
microfilariae appear in the blood mainly at night time
when mosquitoes bite. Some of these filariae are also
found in cats, dogs and some monkeys.

2. Filaria causing Calabar Swellings (*Loa*) is carried by
a cattle fly called Chrysops with dappled wings. The
adult male and female worms wander about the body
and often appear under the skin causing puffy swellings
which only last for a few days. But they may also cause
bad skin irritation generally over the back. They may
also be seen crossing the white of the eye under the thin
membrane called the conjunctiva. They are a little
thicker than the Bancrofti filaria and their microfilariae
are found in the blood mainly in the day when the flies
bite. They are also found in some monkeys.

3. Filaria causing blindness (*Onchocerca*) is carried by a
midge called Phlebotomus which breed in fast running
clear streams. Where these midges abound the people
often quit the area because their bites are so irritating.
The adults live in the small nodules found under the
skin over the ribs and hips and elsewhere. Their
microfilariae swarm just under the skin which becomes
thickened and very itchy. If nodules occur on the
scalp the microfilariae from them may irritate the eyes
and cause blindness.

Prevention consists in insect control measures and
the wearing of clothing to avoid getting bitten.
Treatment. Go to the doctor.

2. YELLOW FEVER

This is another disease carried by the mosquito. Yellow fever occurs around the Gulf of Mexico, in South America, and in Equatorial Africa. Monkeys in these regions are found to suffer from it, and their own special mosquitoes in the forest canopy keep the disease going. Human beings living close to wild monkeys may get infected, and man's own domestic mosquitoes can then spread it and cause serious epidemics.

Its Cause.—The germ is a virus, and human infection is due to the " Tiger " mosquito called Aëdes. When

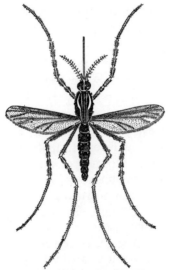

Fig. 45.—Aëdes or Tiger Mosquito.

it gets into the mosquito's stomach the germ takes twelve days before it is ready to cause the disease in another person.

The Disease.—The main sign of yellow fever is that the skin and eyes of the patient become yellow owing to bile getting into the blood; it is this yellow appearance that gives the fever its name. In a bad attack the patient vomits black stuff, the kidneys are affected, and a lot of bleeding takes place under the skin. The disease is very fatal.

Prevention of Yellow Fever.—As in the case of malaria and filaria we can prevent this deadly disease by protecting ourselves from mosquitoes. The " Tiger " mosquito is easy to recognize, for it gets its name " tiger " from its markings. Its legs and body are striped with white. It is very dark, and on its back can be seen markings like a lyre or harp.

Unlike most other mosquitoes tiger mosquitoes bite during the day as well as the night. They are " domestic breeders ", that is, they like to lay their eggs on water in or near a house. They will breed on board ship and in this way can carry the disease about from port to port.

Success of Measures against Yellow Fever.—In the island of Cuba, every year before 1901, about 500 people used to die of yellow fever. In that year the Governor made war against mosquitoes and their larvæ. He put in force the methods we have described in the chapter on Prevention of Malaria. The next year only five people died of yellow fever, and since then Cuba has been free of the disease.

The great French engineer de Lesseps, who made the Suez Canal, tried to cut a canal through the isthmus of Panama. The country was so full of infected mosquitoes that 50,000 of the workmen died of malaria or yellow fever and the work had to be given up. Later on American engineers attempted the task. But this time they fought the mosquitoes first and cleared them out of the Panama canal zone. When this was done they soon cut the canal. Very few of the workmen were sick, and the district is now quite healthy.

Vaccination.—In 1935 American doctors working in Ghana found a man named Asibi suffering from yellow fever. They inoculated monkeys with his blood, and from them they made a vaccine which has proved to be very good in preventing the disease; and Asibi 17D vaccine is still largely used. Asibi was awarded a civil pension as a reward for the good he has done to mankind without knowing it!

Vaccination is done for people going into dangerous yellow fever areas, especially if they are to fly into Asia afterwards. This stops them from spreading the disease into Asia, where it has been prevented until now. Mosquitoes are prevented from travelling in aeroplanes for the same reason; this is done by spraying the aircraft at the aerodromes.

3. DENGUE

A much commoner fever carried by Aëdes is called dengue. Though sometimes painful and weakening, it only lasts a few days and is never fatal. It disappears when " Tiger " mosquitoes are kept down.

4. RELAPSING FEVER AND TYPHUS

As its name implies, *relapsing fever* consists of a series of high fevers. These fevers last for a few days and then go down. After a few days they come again. It is widespread and due to small wavy germs carried not by the mosquito but by *Lice* and *Ticks*. The relapsing fever which is common in Central Africa is caused by the tick, but in Europe and Asia by lice. *Typhus* is another fever carried by lice. It is commoner in temperate than tropical parts. *Tick typhus* occurs in India; grass mites carry *scrub typhus* in Malaya and Japan; there is also a *flea typhus* in some towns.

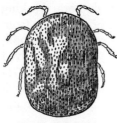

Fig. 46.—A Soft Tick.
(Four times natural size)

Ticks distend themselves with blood; drop off and hide in cracks or holes in the hut near the hearth, where they lay their eggs. After a time the eggs hatch and the little larvæ crawl about; they can also bite and drink blood; they then go underground again and soon change into full-grown ticks, either male or female.

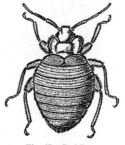

Fig. 47.—Bed Bug.
(Four times natural size)

Bed Bugs lead a similar life, but prefer to hide in seams of hard material, mosquito nets, cracks in wood, or books, and lay their eggs there.

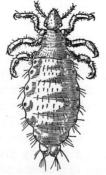

Fig. 48.—The Body-louse.
(Six times natural size.)

Lice live still nearer to us: the *head-louse* and *pubic* or *crab-louse* actually stay on the body and stick their eggs (*nits*) on the hairs; the *body-louse* lives in the clothes, attaching its nits to the fibres of these.

Prevention.—Lice can be dealt with by shaving the hairs or boiling the clothes which are harbouring them. Doctors and sanitary inspectors use D.D.T. or gammexane which kill lice and other insect parasites. If the room is a mud one fill up all cracks with mud to which has been added some insect poison, such as D.D.T. or gammexane.

If you cannot obtain these new medicines, you can destroy bugs and probably ticks with soap. Strong soap solution kills those bugs which it touches and keeps others away. The attack may be made by scrubbing and painting. As the eggs are not easy to kill, it must be made weekly, not only until we think there are no more bugs but *three times after the last bug or tick has been biting*.

When sleeping in an untreated house, we can avoid ticks by sleeping off the ground on some kind of bedstead. Wooden beds should be rubbed with vaseline. By washing and sunning our blankets regularly, we kill yet more of the larvæ.

5. SLEEPING SICKNESS

This disease is one which is confined to Africa. In 1903 there was a great epidemic of it among the people living round the shores of Lake Victoria in Central Africa. Nearly a quarter of a million of them died, and in the blood of the victims were found small parasites named *Trypanosomes*. These parasites are little fish-like bodies which have a tail or whip attached to them. It was afterwards proved by Sir David Bruce that these germs were introduced into the human body by the bite of the tsetse fly. In several parts of Africa a similar disease attacks horses and cattle and causes serious losses to farmers.

The Disease.—The name " Sleeping Sickness " was given because of the sleepy condition into which patients fall during the last stages of the disease. At first there is fever with a skin rash. Then the glands of the neck swell. A persistent headache usually comes on soon. Later—it may be months after—the habits of the man begin to change. He becomes dull, lazy, and careless. Soon his mind becomes clouded and he cannot answer questions properly. The last stage arrives

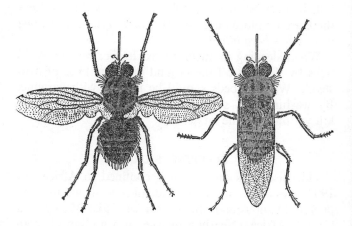

Fig. 49.—The Tsetse Fly. (About three times natural size.)

when he begins to sleep a great deal, and finally he dies.

East African sleeping sickness comes on more quickly. All these stages may take only a few days; or the patient may go mad instead of sleepy.

Prevention of Sleeping Sickness.—We can easily see that the prevention of the disease is a question of avoiding tsetse flies. No one would get it if the flies were all destroyed or avoided.

The tsetse fly is larger than the house-fly and has a long proboscis sticking out of its head. It is very persistent in its attack on man. At rest it closes its wings like a pair of scissors.

The fly usually breeds in bushes close to water. It does not lay eggs but gives birth to larvæ which it drops on the ground. These soon turn into pupæ from which the complete fly emerges. The fly itself bites chiefly during the daytime and does not as a rule travel far from water. Some kinds of tsetse fly, however, act in the opposite way and seek the open country. This is specially true of the ones that carry East African or Rhodesian sleeping sickness. If one has to pass through a country where there is a lot of sleeping sickness it is wise to observe the following rules:

1. Travel early in the morning, or if possible at night, to avoid the flies.
2. Protect the body by wearing long trousers, long sleeves, and a neckerchief.
3. Keep away from water as much as possible.
4. Avoid the areas where tsetse are known to be.

Those who have to live in a country where there is sleeping sickness should see that the bush is cleared around water for at least 100 yards, and around the village or house for 300 yards. Ask the inspectors which trees to cut down in your area. But in spite of all precautions sometimes the only remedy is to move the village right away from the tsetse-fly district.

To-day this disease is being specially studied and successful remedies have been introduced. Finding and treating patients in the glandular stage is one of the best ways of preventing it from spreading.

An injection of a drug called Pentamidine can be given every six months and protects against infection.

6. PLAGUE

The last insect-borne disease we shall consider is Plague. It has spread from its original home (China) to almost every country in the world. It is probably always present in some part of India and in Africa. Probably no other disease has caused so many deaths as plague. The " Black Death ", which destroyed a great part of the population of England and Europe in the fourteenth century and at varying intervals later, is only plague under another name.

The Disease.—There are three forms: Bubonic, Pneumonic and Septicæmic.

(1) *Bubonic plague* is characterized by swellings (buboes) of the lymphatic glands in the groin, the armpits and the neck. There is fever and the patient looks desperately ill. This form is neither so fatal nor so infectious as (2) and (3); it is passed on by the flea.

(2) *Pneumonic plague* is a rarer variety in which the germ attacks the lungs. It is extremely fatal and almost every patient dies in three to four days. This form is very infectious. The sputum, or spit, of the sufferer is full of the plague bacillus and anyone in the same room with him is likely to get the disease. It is not insect-borne.

(3) *Septicæmic plague.*—Here the germs from the flea get into the human blood-stream and excreta. This variety is extremely fatal. Modern treatments are now curing a good many cases even of these bad kinds of plague.

Cause.—Plague reaches us from rats. In countries where the disease is common, if a great number of rats have died, an outbreak of plague nearly always follows.

It is really a *rat disease* and human beings get the disease from them, or from other rodents. Fleas are the carriers. The fleas which live on the body of an infected rat soon become infected themselves. When the rat dies the fleas leave its body and seek food elsewhere. If they bite a man the germ passes into his body and he gets the disease. This is the usual way in which plague is spread. We have seen, however, that in the pneumonic and septicæmic forms the disease may be spread by a patient's breath and sputum or his excreta.

Prevention of Plague.—(1) To prevent the spread of the disease we must obviously get rid of all the rats. If they are present in a house they must be attacked by poison and traps. The house itself should be rat-proof, and above all should be very clean. Rats will only infest houses where they can get food and drink, and if all food is well guarded by safes and tins, and the kitchen and yard kept clean, they will go elsewhere. Even bamboo houses can be made more or less rat-proof. Where bamboo is much used, as in Indonesia, sanitary experts will be able to advise about these methods.

(2) Another measure is to avoid fleas. The house should be scrupulously clean and kept free from insects (see page 146). Fleas can only jump a few inches, so if one sleeps off the floor on a clean bed there is little danger of being bitten at night.

(3) Inoculation. Fortunately there is vaccine which will protect from plague. As its full effect only lasts from six to nine months, the inoculation should be given to as many people as possible each time plague attacks their town.

(4) Drug prevention. There are medicines (" sulpha

drugs ") which can prevent infection if taken by contacts.

Streptomycin, the drug much used against tuberculosis, is also a good cure for plague.

Chapter 17

WATER-BORNE DISEASES

It is usual to call Dysentery, Cholera and Typhoid Fever water-borne diseases; they are common tropical diseases, though happily cholera and typhoid are not common to all parts. The last two are certainly caused by a contaminated water supply, but it is doubtful whether this is the main cause of dysentery. Dysentery is more a hand-borne or fly-borne than a water-borne disease and is often passed on by human carriers. Let us consider each of them briefly.

THE DYSENTERIES

These are diseases which attack the large bowel. They are caused in the main by two organisms—(a) a bacillus which gives rise to *Bacillary Dysentery*, and (b) a small animal parasite (amœba) which causes *Amœbic Dysentery*. Bad diarrhœa may be brought on by drinking dirty water, even if no special germ be present.

Although dysentery is not one of the most fatal of diseases it has bad after-effects, and as soon as the disease makes its appearance it should be attended to. Neglected dysentery may render a person's life miserable; amœbic dysentery may lead to abscess of the liver—a serious complaint.

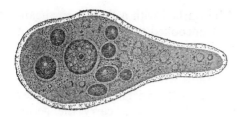

Fig. 50a.—Dysentery Amœba feeding on red blood cells.

Fig. 50b.—Amœbic cyst in stool spreads infection.

The Disease.—Dysentery usually begins by an attack of diarrhœa, but after a few hours or perhaps days the desire to go to stool becomes stronger and may be almost continuous. The stools become scanty and mixed with blood and slime. The tongue becomes coated and the patient loses appetite and gets very weak.

Treatment.—Dysentery needs treatment by a doctor, but until he comes the patient should be kept in bed. Dysentery can usually be cured (*a*) on a light liquid diet, (*b*) the " sulpha " drugs in tablets are used for bacillary dysentery, but a dose of castor oil is a good start. Amœbic dysentery needs injections and other treatment. If a dysentery does not clear up in a few days it is probably amœbic.

Prevention.—(1) The fæces from patients suffering from the disease are dangerous, and it is important to cover them so that flies and other insects cannot get on to them. They should be mixed with disinfectant and then burned or buried. Again, the house and its surroundings must be kept clean, so that flies may not breed there.

(2) Water should always be boiled before drinking during epidemics. If milk is obtained fresh from cows or goats it should likewise be boiled before use.

(3) Fruit should be washed with a little permanganate. Salads (made of uncooked vegetables) should not be eaten during epidemics of dysentery as they are a common source of infection. All food should be covered and kept in safes which are insect-proof.

(4) Some people (called " carriers "), although they are not suffering from the disease, carry the germs in their bowels, and unless the latrines are kept clean and the excreta well covered, flies are likely to carry the germs to food in the house.

(5) No one should touch other people's food, or even their own, unless they have just washed their hands. Especially after going to the W.C., where some carrier may have left germs on the seat, chain or door-handle, we must wash. Until the doctor has passed him free from dysentery, the patient must not work in the kitchen; he may be a carrier.

CHOLERA

Cholera is one of the most deadly of tropical diseases. Its chief home is India but it can be carried to any warm country by carriers. The germ is a microbe shaped like a comma, and this gets into water or milk or on food, and when swallowed by a person brings on the disease. The chief way in which water becomes infected with the germ is by means of the fæces of cholera patients. We have seen, in studying water supply, how important it is that wells should not be near latrines and that the patients' clothes should not be washed near the source of drinking water. We now see that in countries where cholera is found this is doubly important. There has been none in Tropical Africa for a very long time.

The Disease.—Cholera has three stages. (1) *Diarrhœa* (for five to six hours), in which the stools become almost like water. The patient vomits and becomes intensely thirsty. (2) *Collapse* (for two to twenty-four hours), during which the patient becomes very cold. Death often takes place during this stage but the doctor can save life by saline injection. (3) *Recovery*, which takes place in from about twelve to twenty-four hours. The patient becomes warmer and sleeps.

Prevention.—(1) The only way in which the disease can be prevented is to have a pure water supply, and this should be the aim of every town. (2) Should the disease be about, we must use **all** the precautions mentioned in the section on Dysentery. Everything to do with food should be scrupulously clean—plates, basins, pots, should be washed in boiling water. Flies should be attacked in every way possible. Milk and water should be boiled and no raw vegetables eaten. The excreta (stools and urine) of the patient must be disinfected and safely disposed of.

Inoculation can protect against cholera for a short time.

TYPHOID OR ENTERIC

This is a disease which attacks young people rather than old. It occurs in all parts of the world. It is a water-borne disease and, as in the cases of dysentery and cholera, is spread by germs from fæces reaching our food or drink. Even slightly soiled hands can be responsible; thus a common cause of epidemics of typhoid is eating ice-cream made by a typhoid carrier.

Typhoid is due to a germ which enters the mouth and then breeds in the bowel. The first trouble in typhoid is a bad headache; the temperature rises day after day and malaria treatment does not bring it down. Typhoid fever is a disease which needs very careful nursing if the proper treatment is not available.

Owing to the formation of ulcers in the bowels, as the patient gets better he becomes very hungry. But it is dangerous for him to eat hard food because the walls of the bowel are very weak and might easily be pierced, which would cause death. There is now a medicine which cures typhoid in a few days; but it has to be given by a doctor. It is called chloramphenicol.

Paratyphoid fever is like typhoid fever, but is usually not so serious.

Prevention.—Prevention consists in these seven steps:

(1) Protect the water supply.
(2) Dispose of urine and stools of sick people and those recently sick.
(3) Fly-proof latrines.
(4) Protect food and drink from flies.
(5) Clean house and yard to prevent fly breeding.
(6) Wash hands before meals and after going to latrine.
(7) Have two injections of the anti-typhoid inoculation called T.A.B. which gives some protection for about two years.

Chapter 18

WORM DISEASES

Worm diseases occur all over the world, and hookworm and roundworm are very common in the tropics. Of 100 boarders examined in a Nigerian school one only was free from them; Indian labourers in Malaya are found to need " worming " every year; and so on.

1. The Roundworm.—This worm looks rather like the common earthworm. In the intestines of men and pigs, they produce a great number of eggs, but these have to leave the body (in the fæces) before they hatch into worms. The eggs can hatch even after becoming dry and being blown about in dust. When they enter the body of a man or pig, the baby worm finds its way out of its shell. It settles in the lung till it is bigger; then it is coughed up and swallowed; it grows into a big worm in the intestines. The larvæ are a common cause of pneumonia or bronchitis in children. They may cause pain and tenderness in the stomach. From time to time, one worm may be passed at latrine, or escape by the nose. The adult worms sometimes block a child's intestines. They are easily expelled with the proper medicine, piperazine.

2. Threadworms.—These are very small white worms which live in the lower part of the bowel. The female lays her eggs outside the anus, and returns into the bowel. Her body being rough, she makes the anus itch. The patient scratches, so that the eggs often lodge beneath children's finger-nails. The child may suck the fingers and so get more of the worms, or may leave some of the eggs on other people's food and so infect them. The doctor or nurse can remove threadworms from the intestine with piperazine. The patient, and his parents and teachers, should keep his nails short and clean.

3. Tapeworms.—These, as their name implies, are like tape in appearance. They are flat and white and in sections joined together. When full grown they are several yards in length. When the eggs in the sections are ready, whole sections pass out of the body at stool. The sections of the worm decay and the eggs are thus set free. These find their way with grass or other food into the stomach of pigs or cattle where they hatch, and the embryo gets into the blood-vessels the animal and finally lodges in a muscle or the liver, where it remains. When this meat is eaten raw the

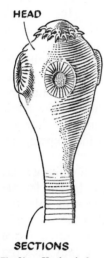

HEAD

SECTIONS

Fig. 51. — Head end of a
Tape-worm. (Magnified.)

embryo grows into a tapeworm. We see therefore that, as in the case of many other parasites, two animals (one may be a man) are required for the life of a tapeworm.

There are several varieties of tapeworm. Sometimes beef has such a worm in it. But, much more often, pigs eat our excrement and get the worms. Hence we should avoid eating unsound meat, especially pork. In any case meat should be thoroughly cooked to kill any worms which may possibly be present. In towns all meat sold publicly ought to be inspected, and if worms are found it should be destroyed. Beef tapeworms, however, rarely cause serious trouble. People

with such worms are usually thin. The proper medicine will expel them, either dichlorophen or yomesan.

4. Hookworm.—This is a worm which inhabits the duodenum. It is a short worm with hooks on the mouth by which it attaches itself to the bowel. Even when passed after treatment it is very difficult to see. It drinks blood from the patient; if there are many hundreds present he soon suffers from anæmia, especially if the diet is poor and lacks iron It causes dullness in school and unfitness for hard work, weakness, pallor and palpitation.

Spread.—The worm lays eggs in the patient's intestine and these are excreted by him. These eggs soon hatch out, the hookworm larvæ find their way into soft earth or mud, and from there they find entrance into the body of another person, because the larva is able to pass through the skin into the blood and

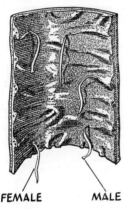

FEMALE   MALE

Fig. 52.—The Hookworm attached to bowel. (Natural size.)

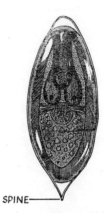

SPINE

Fig. 53.—Spined Egg of a Fluke. (Highly magnified.)

reaches the lungs and finally the bowel. Walking with bare feet in mud, especially near a shallow earth latrine, may thus give one the disease.

It can easily be cured by alcopar or other medicines, plus iron, but is easily caught again. To avoid getting it one should not walk barefoot in damp places in or near villages where people may have used the bush or river as a latrine.

5. Flukes.—In some parts of Asia and Africa there are several kinds of worms called " flukes ". They may inhabit the *blood, liver, bowel* or *lung* in man, and give rise to serious disease. One which is very common in man is *Bilharzia*. It lays its eggs in the veins of the bladder or bowel of its victim. These eggs then work their way into the bladder or bowel and cause bleeding. The blood passes out with the urine or fæces and the man becomes pale and weak. The eggs hatch in water; the larva swims about until it finds a certain water snail. It enters the body of the snail and there changes and produces other young ones. These

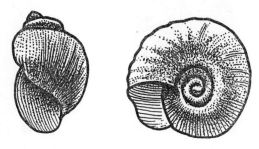

Fig. 54.—Bilharzia-carrying Snails.

escape from the snail into the water and wait for a chance to enter the body of man again. They pierce the skin, as in the case of the hookworm, when a person with bare legs wades in the water. They soon find their way to the veins and cause the disease. It is also called *Schistosomiasis*. Better drugs are now being made to cure it by injection.

Prevention.—Take care not to bathe in any water in places where fluke disease is known to be. Latrine discipline is most important in bilharzia areas.

6. Guinea-Worm.—This disease is found in West Africa, Egypt, Uganda, Arabia and India, and resembles bilharzia in that the worm requires a water animal to complete its life-cycle. The worm grows to 2 or 3 feet long under the skin, generally of the leg. At a spot near the foot, it forms a sore. From this sore, small embryos, or baby worms, escape when the patient stands in water. If they are then eaten by a water-flea (the Cyclops), they undergo changes to fit them for life in our bodies.

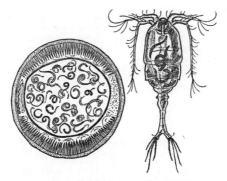

Fig. 55.—(Left) Guinea-Worm embryos and (right) Cyclops water flea. (Highly magnified.)

These fleas are very small and may easily be swallowed by human beings in drinking water. When this happens, the insect is killed by the digestive juices of the stomach and the little worms are liberated. After about nine months the worm appears forming a sore and the whole process begins again.

Treatment of Guinea-Worm.

(1) Protect the worm from injury and bathe the parts frequently with water. This causes it to discharge its embryos. In 2 or 3 weeks it dies, turns white and starts to slide out.

(2) Wind on a small stick every day the inch or two of dead worm which slides out easily. Paint the wound with acriflavine. Bandage the stick and the worm on to the leg. Do not pull, because, if the worm breaks, germs get into the flesh; these may cause abscesses or bad fever.

Doctors can get the worm out a little sooner by injecting drugs which kill it.

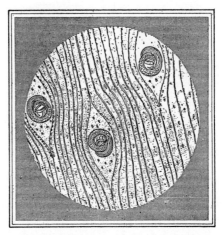

Fig. 56.—Trichina Worm in its Bag in a Muscle. (Highly magnified.)

7. Trichinæ.—These worms are very small, and their lives, which are spent entirely within the bodies of animals or men, may be divided into two parts: (*a*) that spent in the *intestines*, and (*b*) that spent in the *muscles*. In (*a*) the worms breed thousands of embryos which pierce the walls of the blood-vessels and are carried by the blood-stream into the muscles, where they coil up and become enclosed in little bags. Here, stage (*b*), they lie and do not change again. These worms are often found in the flesh of the pig and if a man eats the pork raw, or not cooked enough, the worms get into his stomach where they breed. They cause sharp diarrhœa, and then pass to his muscles, causing fever and pain.

Prevention.—We can easily prevent these worms from doing harm by cooking our meat thoroughly. As far as man is concerned only the pig is likely to give him this worm, and so we should see that any pork we eat is properly inspected and well cooked; boiling will kill any worms in it if the pork is cut up small.

Summary.—We have seen that worms can enter our bodies in four ways:

1. In our drinking-water. (Guinea-worm and possibly Roundworm and Threadworm.)

2. When we eat uncooked or half-cooked meat, especially pork. (Tapeworm and Trichinæ.)

3. When we bathe in fresh water (Flukes), or walk barefoot on mud. (Hookworms.)

4. From dirt on our fingers or food, or blowing about. (Roundworm and Threadworm.)

We can therefore protect ourselves from these worm diseases by—

1. Having pure drinking-water.

2. Cooking our meat well, and seeing that any uncooked food we eat is well washed.

3. By avoiding mud and dirty water.

4. By having very short clean nails and washing well before handling or eating food.

Notice also that to prevent the spread of worm diseases (as well as of many other diseases) *all excreta should be buried away from dwelling-places and wells.*

Babies must be taught to use a chamber pot, and the latrine house must be kept clear of excreta.

Cleaning after Stool.—Water is better than paper for cleaning the anus. Remember this and keep it up. Do not adopt European habits unless they are better than your national ones. The hands must be washed with soap and water after stool, whether paper or water is used for cleaning the anus.

Pigs and Disease.—Three bad worms come from pigs. So we are better without pigs unless we can keep them in sties away from our villages, and give them proper food. Pigs are also blamed for spreading scabies and jiggers. Cattle, goats and sheep hardly give us any serious worms, and are quite safe if the meat from them is well cooked.

Chapter 19

CONTACT DISEASES (CONTAGIOUS)

Many germs or parasites which come into contact with the skin can grow in it and cause such conditions as septic sores or the itch. Others can get through the skin, by a wound or the bite of an animal, and grow in the blood, causing general diseases like Yaws or lock-jaw.

SEPTIC SORES

These are common where people wear little clothing to protect them, or in those who are often in close contact with each other, like school children. The scabs

must be cleaned off and antiseptic paint or ointment
put on. They should be covered to prevent scratching
and flies.

ULCERS

Ulcers are large open sores. In one kind called the
Tropical ulcer the edges are very hard and inflamed
and get quickly eaten away so that the ulcer gets large
and painful and has a foul smelly discharge. These
must be dressed with acriflavine or, better, aureo-
mycine lotion and the patient made to rest up. More
chronic ones are covered with ointment on gauze and
an adhesive plaster.

BOILS AND CARBUNCLES

Boils are due to pus germs getting into the deeper
layers of the skin. They are very painful till they get
ripe and burst, letting out pus and a green core. Do
not squeeze boils, paint some tincture of iodine round
them and then cover with an adhesive plaster. Car-
buncles are like larger boils with more than one head.
It is best to have penicillin before they get too big.

RINGWORM

Ringworms are caused by a mould or fungus which
grows in the skin, most often in the groin (Dhobie's
Itch) or between the toes (Athlete's Foot) or on the
scalp. To avoid them, regular bathing and careful
drying of the skin is important, and the wearing of
loose clothing and sandals without socks. Tincture of
Iodine is a good first aid remedy, but doctors may
order other ointments or drugs. There is a good new
one for ringworm of the scalp, though this condition
goes by itself at the age of puberty. One should be
careful not to use the cap or hat or hair-brush, shoes,
towel or clothing of persons who have got ringworm.

M

THE ITCH OR SCABIES

This skin disease is caused by an *animal* parasite, a small mite about one-fifteenth of an inch long, which can be seen with the naked eye. It burrows into the skin, usually between the fingers, and there the female lays its eggs. These soon hatch and so the mites multiply at a great rate. The itch-mites cause a great deal of irritation and little watery swellings appear on the skin. The disease is contagious and is usually caught by sleeping in the same bed as people already suffering from it.

Treatment.—Wash the part well with hot water and soap. Scabies can best be dealt with by covering the person's body with benzyl benzoate cream or with anti-mite lotion; it should be done three times on successive days, and need not be rubbed in. Wash off after 15 minutes. All the household's clothing and bedding should be aired daily for a week, or boiled. If several members of a household have the itch, the house itself should be thoroughly cleaned; otherwise the disease may come again even if it is cured by treatment.

YAWS

This is another disease which can be passed from person to person by contact. It is well known in the tropics though there is more of it in some parts than in others. The yaws are small swellings with thick scabs, and the discharge from them is infectious. To prevent the spread of this disease the patient should have injections. If not properly treated it may come back in later life, causing big ulcers and painful swellings on bones. It may remain as chronic sores or cracks on the soles of the feet, called " crab yaws ". Injections stop the germ from spreading through the family as it otherwise does. Until the skin is normal, a child with yaws should not sleep with other children, carry them about, or be carried about by them. Clothing also tends to prevent yaws; it is rare in children who wear clothes. But the germ of it can be carried by flies and so get into sores.

LEPROSY OR HANSEN'S DISEASE

This is a very widespread disease. From the earliest times it has been known to be contagious. At one time it was common in Europe but is now practically unknown there. It causes discoloured patches in the skin, either pale or copper coloured in dark skins. Later little lumps or nodules appear, often in the face and ears first. If nerves are attacked there is loss of feeling and weakness of muscles causing paralysis and deformities.

The rod-shaped germ discovered by Hansen is found in the skin and in the discharge from the nose and from some, but by no means all, of the sores. Those with discharging germs should be isolated from other people. A great number of such cases are allowed to mix with people in the market places and streets of most tropical towns. If each bad or infectious case could enter a special village or " colony ", not only would his life be much happier and his disease be relieved, but in the course of a generation the disease would be stamped out. At the present time great progress is being made and there is a treatment for leprosy which can mostly cure it. This does not do away with the need for " colonies "; indeed, it makes it more desirable that every case should be given the chance of being cured. In some countries, people with leprosy can, while they are not spreading the germs, be treated as out-patients. Many of them have thus been fully cured while still living at home, without danger to the rest of the family.

VENEREAL DISEASES

Venereal Diseases (V.D.)—The germs are passed on almost always by sexual contact. That is why they affect first the genital organs or the urinary passage and cause sores or discharges. There are six such diseases but the commonest are gonorrhœa and syphilis.

Gonorrhœa.—Burning pain and white pus in the urinary passage may mean gonorrhœa and need immediate treatment *by a doctor*. Packets or bottles of medicine or unskilled syringing are dangerous. The disease is easy to hide and, in the early stages, fairly easy for the doctor to cure. It causes many sicknesses; and people who have had it are often unable to have children. The worst cases of pus in the eyes are due to this disease. Babies often catch it in the birth canal and may become blind.

Syphilis.—This forms a sore near the urinary passage. Six weeks or so later, a rash occurs. Months or years later, unless the patient has had a full course of injections, other sores occur and many other troubles may follow. The worst effects fall on the children, if any, who may die young, go blind, become insane, or have sick children themselves.

Prevention.—Except for the rare cases where they are sick because of their parents' misbehaviour, if a boy and girl have not had sexual intercourse before they marry, they cannot have venereal disease. Is it possible to live in this ideal way, to practise what is called " continence "? Yes. Many thousands of men and women practise it either for life or until they marry; and then they have children quite normally. The organs of reproduction do *not* need exercise. Like other laws of health, the strength to keep this rule *can* be found.

If people have not got this control over their bodies, there is no medicine which can prevent these diseases with any certainty. In many parts of the tropics, practically everyone who allows his or her body to be abused by " fornication " (sexual union before marriage) has venereal disease. And it is very hard for doctors to prove whether the disease is finished or whether it is infectious and therefore still dangerous.

When married, the man and wife will, of course, keep their marriage vow; breaking it is called " adultery ". If there were no adultery or fornication, V.D. would cease to exist. Still more important, only parents who are loyal to each other have homes in which children can grow up healthy in body and mind. A family may be spoilt for the sake of short-lived pleasures, but good homes are the source of life-long happiness. They also form the back-bone of a healthy national life.

SUMMARY

In our study of the skin and contagious diseases we have once more noticed the *importance of cleanliness*. Especially do we see the importance of clean hands and clothing. In a tropical country, where cotton is the chief material used and where few clothes are worn, there is no excuse for dirty clothing. Clothes can be washed, dried and ironed in a few hours. We should be careful that our bedclothes are clean. All clothes other than woollens should be dried by hanging them in the sun so that air and heat can act on them. Woollens and flannels should be dried out of the sun.

We can see how important it is to wash our hands. Our hands go everywhere and pick up all kinds of dust and dirt. It is not sufficient to bath in the morning and think one is clean for the rest of the day. The hands need washing *several times a day* with soap and water. At least this ought to be done before a meal, for even if we do not eat with our fingers there is always the danger of germs passing from our fingers to our mouths.

Many people, such as Muslims, are very strict about washing before meals. But in some towns one rarely sees a boy wash his hands before eating; he prefers to do this afterwards when his fingers are soiled with food. In view of the danger of spreading disease germs it would be a good thing if " Wash before eating " were made a motto. We should not suck anything which others may have sucked: that is one way throat diseases are caused. Not only must our spoons and cups be clean, but sucked fingers and spoons should be kept out of other people's food. Many people are very careful about this, and all should be.

Chapter 20

MORE TROUBLES FROM ANIMALS AND INSECTS

In this chapter, we shall study some of the sicknesses which we may get from animals and troublesome creatures which we have not described yet, and which we must understand if we are to keep healthy.

LEPTOSPIROSIS (INFECTIVE JAUNDICE)

Yellow jaundice has many causes. One is the rare disease Yellow Fever (mosquito-borne), another is caused by a small virus germ which attacks the liver, and a third is Leptospirosis. Leptospires are small corkscrew-shaped germs which are found normally in the kidneys of rats, small field mice and also of dogs.

If one bathes or walks in water or damp earth fouled by these animals, the leptospires may get in through a scratch or a small sore, or even through the membrane of the eyes and mouth.

A few days afterwards the patient may get a bad. headache and muscle pains and high fever. Later the yellow jaundice appears owing to damage done to the liver. The germs also attack the membranes round the brain and the disease is often fatal. Penicillin may help to cure it. People working in rat-infested water or sewers or slaughter houses must wear rubber boots and gloves to protect themselves. A preventive vaccine can be used.

TETANUS OR LOCKJAW

This disease can occur wherever horses, or even cattle, have been. It is caused by a germ in their droppings which enters the flesh through a wound and produces a poison. This acts on the nervous system, causing stiffness of the muscles, notably those of the jaws. It often causes death. Occasionally it attacks newly born babies, causing fatal fits. The germ of tetanus lives in the soil, especially ground which has been cultivated, and on roads where horse manure is found.

Prevention.—The disease may be prevented as follows:

1. By seeing that any *slight* wound or scratch is well washed with antiseptic and bound up. This is to prevent any tetanus or other germs from entering the body. A possible source of tetanus is the jigger wound (see page 175), or old ulcers of the leg.

Again, no dirt must be allowed to touch the newly born baby's cord, which must be cut with a boiled instrument and wrapped in sterile dressings.

2. If we get a *deep* wound it is most important that it should be well washed with acriflavine lotion,

especially if earth has got in. Such wounds are commonly got on farms, usually on the feet or legs.

3. Deep wounds should be taken immediately to a doctor or hospital. Hundreds of children and adults die in tropical towns yearly as a result of this disease, so it is impossible to be too careful. There is an *Anti-Tetanus Serum* which, if injected early enough, prevents the disease. It may cure a mild case of tetanus, but it may fail; if given in time, however, it always prevents the disease from starting. During recent wars this serum saved the lives of hundreds of thousands of soldiers who were in danger of tetanus owing to wounds. This " A.T.S." only protects for a few weeks.

4. People who are in special danger of wounds, such as soldiers, are now given an antitoxin; then they cannot have tetanus. Babies who attend welfare clinics are nowadays being given a course of three injections of this. It is called *tetanus toxoid*. It is most important that you report to the hospital for injections when you get a dirty wound, so that you may not develop tetanus.

ANIMAL BITES

1. Dogs, Cats and other Animals.—The bites of dogs or other animals are most dangerous when the animal is itself developing a disease called *Rabies*. If the dog is known to us we can sometimes tell if it has rabies because is is mad; but any dog which bites us must be caught, kept tied up, and properly fed to see if it is beginning to be ill. If it does seem ill or if it dies, the person bitten must go to a doctor, *however slight the wound is*. If the dog dies or is killed, its body must be sent to the doctor as well.

If after ten days the dog is still alive and well, there is nothing to fear, as it is not suffering from rabies. If, however, it seems ill in a few days the doctor will advise what to do. Rabies can be prevented if the patient is treated before any sign of it is present. Once it has started, every case is fatal. Prevention is by inoculations and other treatment which lasts about 3 weeks.

This wonderful discovery is due to a French chemist, Louis Pasteur. He was so horrified to see people dying of rabies that he determined to find the answer. The inoculation was first thought to be very dangerous, and as Pasteur was not a doctor he was running a great risk in using it. But his patients, if they were injected in time, did not develop rabies.

Treatment.—The wound cannot be freed of rabies by any treatment, however strong. So it should just be washed thoroughly with permanganate or acriflavine.

Prevention.—It is not easy to prevent oneself from being bitten by a dog, but it is possible to get rid of all mad dogs in a town or district. Dogs only have rabies after having been bitten by another dog which has rabies. If, therefore, all dogs in a district are muzzled for a few months no dog can be so bitten. Any unowned or unmuzzled dogs should be destroyed by the authorities. There are now no mad dogs to be found in Britain. Rabies is unknown too in Australia, and in Papua and some other islands. The disease could only occur there if a dog suffering from it were to be brought in. This is guarded against by the authorities, and severe punishment is given to people who try to get their dogs into the country without " quarantine " for rabies.

Rabies in dogs can also be prevented by the use of injections. Some countries make it a law that all dogs be inoculated against rabies before they are licensed.

2. Snake-Bite.—Not all snakes are poisonous; indeed, the majority are non-poisonous; but this does not help us in case of snake-bite unless we know the snake to be of a harmless species. Snake-bite demands immediate treatment, and if we wait for symptoms to see if a bite is poisonous we shall probably be too late.

A bite from a poisonous snake shows two red punctures where the poison fangs have entered. Whereas, if one sees many punctures, perhaps in two rows, the snake is probably non-poisonous.

Treatment.—(1) If possible take the patient to a doctor for injection treatment. But before starting—

(2) For a hand or forearm bite, tie the upper arm tightly with a rubber tube, bandage or small padded cord. For a finger or toe, tie its base. For foot or calf, tie in the middle of the thigh. The object of this is to prevent the blood from the poisoned part getting into the blood stream and so poisoning the whole body. This must be *done at once* or it will be too late. Do not lose your head. Even if the snake was a poisonous one perhaps it may have injected only a little poison.

(3) After the limb has been tied, the wound ought to be treated. Usually the flesh around the punctures is cut very freely so as to allow the poisoned blood to flow out. The skin must be wiped before cutting; there may be snake poison on it.

(4) The wound may be sucked. There is no danger in snake poison being taken into the mouth and spat out if there are no cuts on the lips or sides of the mouth. The mouth must afterwards be washed out.

(5) The wound should be washed with soapy water, or potassium permanganate solution can be used. It seldom happens, however, that we have these things handy, and so the tying, cutting and sucking are all that we can do. There are sharp knives to be obtained, called " snake knives ", which have the crystals of permanganate kept in the handle so as to be ready for

immediate use, and one of these should be carried in a snake-infested district. The tight bandage must be released after 20 minutes or it may strangle the limb.

After-treatment: (1) Patient to rest lying down, no movement of limb which must be kept cool with wet cloth or an ice pack over the wound to prevent poison spreading.

(2) If the patient stops breathing, commence artificial respiration (see pages 224–25) and keep it up for a long time, as the poison is continually leaving the body by the sweat and urine and he may survive.

Prevention.—(1) Always wear boots in a snake-infested district. Even hard shoes are a help, because snakes hear them and keep out of the way.

(2) Wear puttees. Snakes rarely bite above the knee.

(3) Carry a strong stick.

INSECT BITES AND STINGS

These bites are rarely serious but may be very painful. We are liable to be bitten by a great number of insects in the tropics, and the effect is usually a certain amount of pain and swelling. If there is a bee's sting left in the wound, it must be removed. The bites of ants, sandflies, mosquitoes, spiders, centipedes or wasps are relieved by applying some alkali such as a blue bag, carbonate of soda or ammonia to the place. Lightly scratching into it some strong soap often stops it itching; such soap is alkaline. (But of course germs from the fingers may enter and cause trouble.) Scorpion stings are extremely painful, but not dangerous. Reassure the patient, and bathe the bitten limb in hot water.

INSECT PARASITES

1. The Jigger or Sand Flea.—This is an African insect which has also spread to India. It attacks

the feet and toes. The female burrows into the skin
and swells up, causing tenderness and irritation. The
body of the jigger is seen under the skin as a black
dot. The eggs, when ripe, develop into fresh jiggers
in dust or dry sand.

To remove a jigger:

(1) Take a safety pin or needle (*not too sharp*) and
hold its point in a flame for a few seconds.

(2) Press back the skin around the black dot and
gradually work the jigger out of its hole, being careful
not to break the bag containing the eggs.

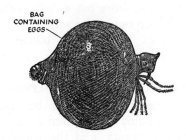

Fig. 57.—The Female Jigger, about five times natural size.

(3) Burn the jigger and eggs in a flame.

(4) Wash out the hole with some strong antiseptic
(iodine or acriflavine) and bind it up till healed so as
not to let dirt get into the hole. Deaths from tetanus
are said to have occurred as a result of the germ getting
into a jigger hole. If jiggers are not removed they may
cause ulcers which sometimes cripple the foot.

Prevention.—Jiggers hatch only on dry floors. Any
house or school known to be infested with them
has only to be thoroughly washed a few times, say
twice a week, and there will be no more trouble. If
a village is badly infested, the children in school should

be made to examine each other's feet every couple of days. D.D.T. spraying kills jiggers.

2. The Tumbu Fly of Africa also hatches in sand or earth. The larva pierces the skin of the arm or buttock. When small, it can be squeezed out; when it is larger, pus comes from the hole; then the maggot must be left to come out by itself or helped out by the doctor.

THE HOUSE-FLY

We have mentioned flies before because of their dirty habits. They settle on all the dirtiest things they can find and then come on to our tables and food. Their way of eating is to vomit some of the juice in their stomach on to the sugar or rice and then suck it back again. So, as they have some germs in their stomach, many germs remain on our food.

Flies' legs are hairy and these hairs can also carry a lot of germs, so any food on which a fly has been sitting is sure to have germs on it. When there is any dysentery in the village, house-flies often carry the germs and leave them on our food.

What can we do if there are too many flies in our compound or in our village? We can, of course, keep all our food covered up except when we are preparing or eating it. We can kill a great many of the flies with fly-swats or even with our hands. But the best method of all is to attack them, as we attack the mosquito, by spraying insecticides in places where the young flies are growing.

The Larva of the House-Fly.—Whenever there are many flies about, it is possible to find where some of them are breeding. Search in the dark places in your compound, turn over manure which is lying about, and go to any place where waste food is rotting. You will then find a rather fat white creature, about as long as a mosquito larva, which crawls about like a caterpillar. This is the house-fly's larva, or maggot.

In the earth near the rubbish or mixed up with it are the pupæ. They are like a large grain of rice with a polished brown skin. If you keep some of them or some of the larvæ in a jar covered with mosquito-netting, flies will come out of them in a few days.

Prevention.—If there is no damp rubbish for the flies to breed in, there will be no flies. Manure and damp rubbish kept in proper compost heaps become so hot that the fly larva dies. Houses and compounds which are clean, and dust bins which are regularly emptied into the incinerator, do not breed flies. If larvæ or pupæ are found in rubbish, it should be burnt. If burning is impossible, deep burying is necessary, at least a foot deep, as larvæ can burrow upwards through the soil. Latrines which are producing flies must be filled in and new and better ones built.

If the places where a fly puts its feet have been covered with a residual insecticide, as was described for other insects on pages 138 and 146, the fly goes away and dies. Spraying is usually done because of the danger of mosquitoes or the trouble caused by biting insects; but it should be done wherever fly-borne diseases like typhoid and dysentery are spreading. Do all you can to encourage your family and neighbours to have it done thoroughly when the health people order it.

SECTION IV

SANITATION

Chapter 21

SEWAGE AND REFUSE

Our studies of various diseases have taught us, above all, the lesson of cleanliness. Without cleanliness we cannot be healthy. But we must not only be personally clean; our towns and villages and our compounds

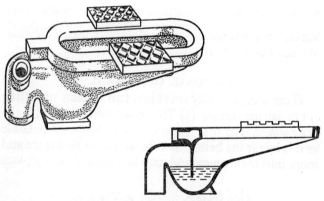

Fig. 58.—A Squatter Pan.

must be clean also. Work done to keep a town or village healthy is called sanitation.

There is need for a system by which the rubbish of a town can be dealt with. Even in villages this matter ought not to be left to ordinary householders to look after, but should be the care of the council, or the local authority aided by Government, who should arrange for the daily cleaning of the village.

Refuse from a town falls naturally into two parts,

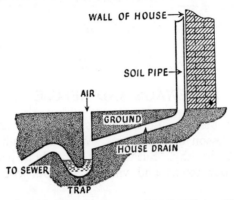

Fig. 59.—Diagram showing Soil Pipe, House Drain and ventilation of Sewer Trap.

latrine refuse (excreta) and ordinary household refuse. We shall consider them in that order.

DISPOSAL OF SEWAGE

There are, generally speaking, two systems of getting rid of latrine refuse. (1) The *water method*, and (2) the *dry method*. The first method is used wherever possible as it is by far the better. It is being introduced more and more into the tropics, and may be installed in any place

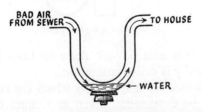

Fig. 60.—Diagram showing a Defective Trap.

with a pipe-line water supply, so a brief account of it is here given. Human excreta mixed with water are called sewage.

WATER-BORNE SEWAGE

Dirty water from baths and kitchens is mixed with

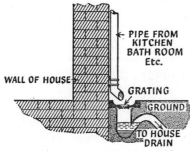

WALL OF HOUSE

← PIPE FROM KITCHEN BATH ROOM Etc.

GRATING

GROUND

TO HOUSE DRAIN

Fig. 61.—Diagram showing Bath Pipe disconnected from Drain.

the sewage and runs into *septic tanks*. In modern towns it goes into a very large pipe which runs under the streets and goes out of the town. This large pipe is called the *Sewer*. Naturally, as it contains all the excreta of the town, it will often have stinking gases in it too.

Traps are devices by which the bad gas from the sewer is prevented from passing upwards into the house. The diagrams show four of them. One is placed between the sewer and the house drain, another between the soil pipe and the pan of the W.C. There are many forms of

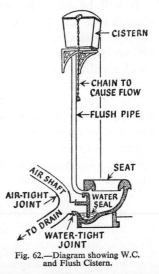

← CISTERN

← CHAIN TO CAUSE FLOW

←FLUSH PIPE

SEAT

AIR SHAFT

AIR-TIGHT JOINT

WATER SEAL

TO DRAIN

WATER-TIGHT JOINT

Fig. 62.—Diagram showing W.C. and Flush Cistern.

N

trap. They are merely bends in the pipe. We must notice with regard to traps—

1. That they are useless unless plenty of water remains in the bends of the pipe as in Fig. 59. Fig. 60 shows how bad air can pass through a trap that has too little water in it.

2. The trap should be easy to reach and be regularly cleaned, as solid matter may stick to the sides of the pipe. Traps should have plugs (as Fig. 60) so that the bend can be cleaned out.

It should be noted that water from baths goes into the house drain (Fig. 61).

The water to wash the pan comes from a flush tank which empties itself when a chain is pulled and then is automatically filled from the main water supply. Fig. 62 gives a general idea of the arrangement. If you have such a cistern you should study it and know how to do simple repairs.

It will be seen that this method of disposing of excreta is a very good one, but it needs a piped water supply. It is also expensive to install. Again, ignorant or careless people may put things into the pan which block the drain. Corn cobs or thick paper, for instance, must not be thrown into lavatories.

The sewage from the town is treated in various ways. Sometimes, after being chemically treated, it is poured into a river or into the sea. More often it is run into *Septic Tanks* in which heavy solids settle and slowly dissolve. The liquid overflows on to filter beds or into other tanks. After filtration, or standing in several tanks, the liquid is almost pure water and is used for irrigating farm land. Disease germs will have died out, provided the germs of decay are allowed free play. This explains the name septic tank: the germs must not be killed by antiseptics, for some germs of disease may escape, and the germs of decay must be allowed to develop. Antiseptics are out of place in the water latrine system. Small septic tanks can also be made for individual compounds or schools, so it is useful to understand them, which you can do by studying the diagram.

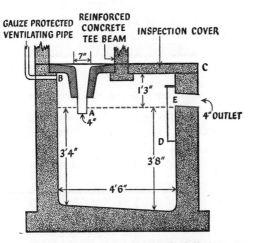

Fig. 63.—Showing the working of a Septic Tank.

Every few months or years the solid matter has to be removed. It is called *sludge*. It is harmless and almost odourless; it is an excellent manure. The tanks must be sealed each time they are opened, otherwise mosquitoes and flies may breed in them.

BUCKET METHODS

These are less used than formerly in the tropics because the water method is more widely available.

1. The Dry Pail System.—This is the most common method. The excreta are passed into pails, and the contents of the pails are removed daily and carted out of the town.

The Latrine.—(1) The latrine should always have a cement floor.

(2) It should be airy and exposed to the rays of the sun.

(3) It should be protected from rain.

(4) The pails should be under a frame-work upon which the person should sit. Latrines with buckets can also be made for use in the squatting position; squatting has great advantages but cannot be done cleanly on a seat.

(5) Unless the pail has a fly-proof lid, there should be ashes, wood shavings or earth available to throw over the excreta. This will keep flies off it and help to prevent the spread of disease.

(6) The pails should be scrubbed out at least once

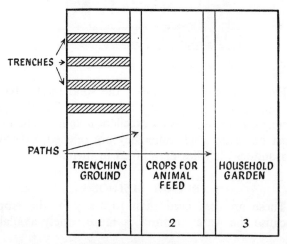

Fig. 64.—Trenching Ground.

The trenches are about eighteen inches deep and just a little wider than the sanitary pail. The plots are changed in rotation, i.e. one year a plot will be trenched, the next year it will have animal crops, and the third year household crops.

a week and put in the sun. The wooden seat likewise should be scrubbed and aired.

Disposal of Excreta.—This varies accordingly to the conditions.

Trenching is used in country districts. A large piece of land is set apart as disposal land. On this land trenches are dug into which the refuse is put, and covered with a layer of earth. It is found that in time the fæces are quite changed and turn into rich soil so that good crops can be grown on the disposal ground. Vegetables which are eaten raw should not be grown on trenching grounds. The safest crop is grass for cattle.

If properly supervised this system is quite satisfactory. The great thing is to see (1) that flies cannot get at the excreta, and (2) that the ground is not overloaded. The germs which live on the excreta and work the change do not act deep in the soil, so the trenches must not be more than 18 inches deep. On the other hand, if the excrement is less than 6 or 8 inches below the surface, fly larvæ will be found in it.

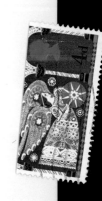

Incineration or Burning.—In this system the excreta are taken outside the town and placed in large furnaces called *incinerators* and burnt. If this method is properly carried out it is the best of the dry methods of sewage disposal, but it needs careful supervision.

The excreta are mixed with dry material (leaves, sawdust or horse-manure) which will absorb the liquid. It is claimed that this system is not only effective but cheap. There is no doubt that this is the best method for the tropics, especially in places where fuel is cheap.

2. The Wet Pail System.—Here the urinals and latrines are provided with disinfectants which are mixed with the excreta. The disinfectants tend to kill any disease germs and to keep off flies. It is claimed that this system reduces greatly the number of flies and therefore keeps down disease. The refuse has, of course, to be buried as in the dry pail system. In some places, where the current takes it out to sea, wet latrine refuse can be dumped outside the breakers.

Though simple in principle there are the following objections to buckets—

(1) Unless the removal of the pails is carefully carried out an opportunity is given for flies to reach the excreta.

(2) Hand removal is expensive and the work is very objectionable.

(3) The cost of iron pails is considerable, and through careless use the life of a sanitary pail is short. Moreover such things are not easily repaired.

(4) This hand removal of excreta is a cause of bad smells, and a source of danger in times of epidemic.

DIRECT BURYING METHODS

We now come to the method which is most used in tropical schools and homes.

1. Deep Pit Latrine, or **Fosse Arabe.**—The hole must be made so deep and covered over so well that it is quite dark at the bottom even when someone raises the lid. Then flies will not breed in it, as they dislike total darkness. Such a hole, 12 or 15 feet deep, and big enough for a man to work in, is a very good latrine. It needs a firm covering of planks which white ant will not eat, or sticks and earth; the hole for sitting or squatting must have a lid. The latrine should have a roof, but it should not be too dark to see if anyone has fouled the woodwork.

2. Bore-hole Latrine.—This is a hole 18 feet deep, made with an 18-inch borer or *auger*. If the soil is suitable and an auger available, this is a splendid type of latrine. It needs covering and roofing like the Fosse Arabe, but this is of course much easier to do. If you have two or more bore-holes, their edges must be at least 18 inches apart.

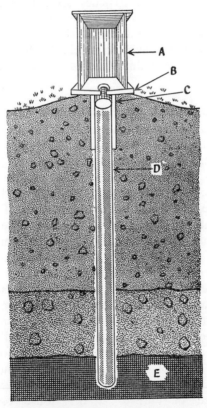

Fig. 65.—A Bore-hole Latrine.
A. Latrine building. B. Floor of cement or wood. C. Large cement pipe, usually not necessary. D. Woven bamboo lining, usually not necessary. E. Water. It does not matter whether the bore-hole reaches water or not.

3. Shallow Trench Latrine or **Midden.**—This is a bad system, only suitable for emergencies. If, for any reason, a deep trench cannot be made, do not try to go as deep as you can. Rather have a trench not more than 5 feet deep, so that everyone can cover his fæces with earth and so keep away smells and flies. Soldiers, when stopping anywhere in the open even for a few hours, dig such trenches, 3 feet long, 3 feet deep and about 9 inches wide, to be used squatting astride. If a seat or roof is put over a shallow latrine, it must not darken the trench too much. Such trenches must be filled in when within 9 inches of the surface.

DISPOSAL OF HOUSEHOLD REFUSE

Each day a certain amount of refuse is produced by every household: waste paper, old rags, empty tins, fruit skins, vegetable peelings and so on. What is to be done with these things? Careless people throw them into the street or into the bush at the back of the house, but this is bad in many ways. The rubbish accumulates and gets wet in the rain. The heat then causes things to rot and give off bad smells. Also decaying meat, fish, fruit or cooked food attracts flies which, in such rubbish, breed. These, as we have seen, are powerful agents for spreading disease. Again, old bottles and tins hold the rain and become breeding places for mosquitoes. It is essential, therefore, that this household refuse should be properly disposed of.

Goats and fowls will eat most of the food refuse. A good deal of what is left can be burned. Indeed all the animal and vegetable matter *ought* to be buried or burned. If the house contains an iron stove burning is easy and saves wood. But in a crowded town where the yards of the houses are too small for livestock, special methods are needed to deal with rubbish. We will discuss this now.

The Dust Bin.—This is a receptacle which holds the household refuse until it is carried away. The bin should be made of iron and should have a fairly closely fitting lid. It should be small, so as to need emptying frequently. It should be cleaned out regularly, and if used only for dry refuse ought to last a long time. *The lid is essential.* It will keep out the rain (and so prevent decay); it will prevent flies from laying eggs in the rubbish.

The custom of storing refuse in baskets or wooden boxes is a bad one. They are difficult to keep flies out of, and difficult to keep clean.

The Rubbish Dump.—In many towns the dust bins are emptied into trucks, and the rubbish taken away by the Town Council, and disposed of at once. This is, of course, the best plan. But sometimes the refuse has to be stored again, and for this purpose rubbish dumps are built. Where the rubbish dump system is used it is essential to the health of the town that the dump be frequently emptied.

The dump must be in an open space away from houses. It must be kept dry. This means that it should have a roof and that it should be raised above the level of the ground in order that rain may not drain into it. Its floor must be waterproof so that dirty water may not sink into the soil and thence into wells. It must be disinfected regularly.

Disposal of the Refuse.—Town Councils have great difficulty in knowing what to do with this refuse. The common practice is to use it to fill in holes and to raise the level of low-lying land. Later on, houses are built on such foundations. In many European towns the refuse is carefully sorted, sometimes with the help of machinery. Most of it is burned in a furnace; the bottles are used for road-making; the fine dust is made into bricks; and iron, rags and paper are put to use again. This method is, however, only possible where factories create a sufficient demand for waste articles.

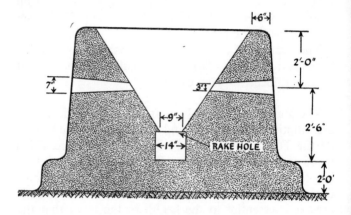

Fig. 66.—Incinerator.

Incineration.—The best plan is, as in the case of sewage, destruction by means of *incinerators*. They should be some distance from the town, otherwise the smell is a great nuisance. After burning, tins and bottles have to be crushed and buried.

Excellent incinerators can be made out of empty 44-gallon oil or petrol drums. Iron stakes driven through form shelves to hold the fire. Even old roofing sheets useless for building can be used to make incinerators in the same way.

But some villages have no iron to spare. Above is a diagram of an incinerator made without bars. Any school which has any difficulty in the disposal of rubbish should build one of these; the only material used is mud. Help may be obtained from Health Inspectors.

There is no doubt that a great deal can be done by the town authorities to make a town healthy. But those most responsible are the *householders themselves*. If the rooms and kitchens and yards of the houses are dirty, the town will be unhealthy however clean the streets may be.

Chapter 22

THE HOUSE AND ITS SURROUNDINGS

People's health depends a good deal on the sort of house they live in, so all houses should be built on sound sanitary principles. Let us see what constitutes a good house.

1. Site and Soil.—A damp house is dangerous to health. All manner of complaints are caused by dampness. Colds are common, and serious diseases such as tuberculosis easily take root, among people living in damp houses.

To be dry a house must be built on a dry soil. Soils are, generally speaking, of two kinds, *porous* and *non-porous*. Examples of porous soils are *gravel, sand, laterite, chalk;* or non-porous, *clay* and *rocks* such as limestone. The best soil to build on is of course the porous. If possible the house should stand on a gentle slope of gravel soil; but even sand and gravel may be damp if they rest on a layer of clay which is only a few feet below. There is sure to be a lot of water resting on the clay. This is known as *ground water*, and during the rains it may rise and cause a house to be damp. If the ground water in a district is less than twelve feet below the surface of the soil, the land ought to be drained before being built on. One method of securing a dry house is to build the house on *piles*. This is especially necessary in swampy districts where the ground water is very near the surface or where floods occur from time to time. Metal caps on piles prevent the house from being attacked by white ants. A more usual method is to make the floor of concrete. This is compulsory in many towns.

2. The Aspect.—This word means whether the house faces North, South, East or West. Sunlight and a certain amount of breeze are essential to health. In the tropics the chief living-rooms should face north or south so as to be cool, but each room ought to get some sunshine daily. Bushes and low trees ought to be cut well away from the windows, and the house ought not to be over-shadowed by other buildings.

3. Construction.—*The rooms* ought to be high and airy with plenty of window space. Building houses with small dark rooms is very bad, for they cannot be well ventilated, and germs breed in dark places.

The walls are usually built of the cheapest material in the district. The chief thing is that they should be damp-proof and white-ant-proof. Mud walls are quite good if they contain a concrete course to prevent white ants getting to the roof. Concrete blocks or bricks are expensive but lasting. They absorb the rain, however, unless rendered waterproof. Whether made of mud, concrete, or brick, exposed walls should be faced with cement or tar except where they are well protected by the roof. The eaves ought to project a good way beyond the walls to shield them from rain. Otherwise even on a dry site the house may be damp.

The roof.—The usual roofing for modern houses in many parts of the tropics is corrugated iron sheets. These are durable and fire-proof, but unless they are lined inside they are apt to make the house very hot. They should always be lined with some non-conducting material such as wood, asbestos, reed or palm matting, or felt. All rooms should have such ceilings, and there should be an air space between the ceiling and the roof. This air space should be ventilated, but at the same time rendered proof against bats and rats by means of netting wire. Grass and leaf roofs are cool but they harbour insects and also are liable to catch fire in the dry season. Tiles, corrugated asbestos, or shingles made of slices of wood (iron-wood or umbrella-tree) are a useful improvement on these thatched roofs, and have been introduced into many villages. They need carpentered rafters, and a few nails. It must be pointed out that water from a shingle roof, like that from thatch, is not good for drinking.

Floors.—A common floor in the tropics is made of mud. When dressed with cow-dung it has a smooth and apparently clean surface. Damp cow-dung, however, attracts flies and breeds germs, hence the system is bad. A better floor is made of concrete. It costs more than some other materials, but it lasts longer and is the most sanitary, being fairly easy to wash. If the corners of the rooms are rounded they are not so likely to harbour dust.

Verandahs.—These are very useful additions to the house. They shield the inner rooms and walls from the glare of the sun and from storms, and provide pleasant sitting-out places in the evening. In districts where mosquitoes abound it is well to have a portion of the verandah rendered mosquito-proof so that it can be used with safety and comfort (see p. 139).

Windows.—These should be *large* and opposite to another window, or at least to a door (see Chapter 3). Lighting of rooms by day depends not only on windows but also on the ceiling: if this is white, the lighting is most pleasant.

4. The Surroundings.—These are important. We have seen that the bush should be cleared right away from the house to allow the air to circulate. Fewer insects will then visit it.

1. The presence of trees is good, so long as they do not cut off the breezes.

2. Marshes and swamps must be avoided or drained as they breed mosquitoes. Some trees, notably eucalyptus or blue gum, are valuable for drying swampy soil.

3. Cesspools and water in the form of lakes, ponds and rivers should not be too near.

4. The house should not be exposed to bad smells such as may rise from rubbish dumps or trenching grounds.

Gardens.—Houses ought to have gardens. These are useful not only on account of the produce they yield but also for the interest they give to the householder. They have a great educative value and give dignity to the house, even though it be a small one. It ought to be the aim of every educated householder to possess a garden which will produce some of the beautiful grasses, shrubs, flowers, vegetables, herbs and fruits which grow so easily in a tropical climate.

Chapter 23

CLIMATE

As the climate of a country has a good deal to do with the health of the inhabitants, we will consider some of the factors which determine the climate of a place.

1. Latitude.—Places near the equator are generally damp with moderate and rather even temperature. The part of the world lying between latitude $23\frac{1}{2}°$ north and $23\frac{1}{2}°$ south of the equator is commonly spoken of as *The Tropics*. Outside these latitudes the sun is never vertically overhead. But just outside them and in big continents, it is far hotter at times than it ever is near the equator.

2. The Seasons.—In tropical latitudes the year is generally divided into two—the wet season and the dry, according to rainfall.

The winds which bring rain from the Indian and Pacific Oceans are called Monsoons. In West Africa, it is the dry season which has its own special wind; this blows from the Sahara desert and is called the Harmattan.

3. Altitude.—The height of a place above sea level affects its climate. The higher it is, the cooler. On an average the temperature falls one degree fahrenheit for every 300 feet we ascend. The air of hilly districts is drier than that of lowlands.

4. Winds.—These affect the climate of a place greatly. Winds which have blown across oceans and seas are damp. Those which have passed over large

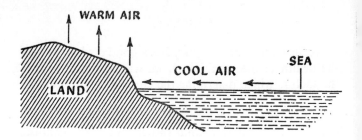

Fig. 67.—Diagram to show Day Sea-breeze.

tracts of land are dry, and either hot or cold according to the season. Countries which get most of their wind from the sea usually have plenty of rain. In the tropics, places near the coast get a sea-breeze during the day and a land-breeze at night. This is because during the day in the tropics, the land is hotter than the sea, so the air above the land is warmer than the air above the sea. This warm air rises (see page 14) and its place is taken by the cool sea air. This forms a sea-breeze (see diagram).

At night the conditions are reversed. The land is cooler than the sea. The actual temperature of the sea hardly changes from day to night but the tem-

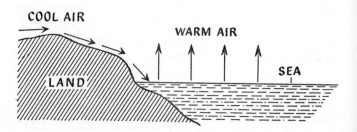

Fig. 68.—Diagram to show Night Land-breeze.

perature of the land changes greatly, and at night the air over the land becomes cold. The warmer air over the sea rises and a land-breeze blows to take its place.

5. Rainfall affects temperature considerably. Where there is an abundant rainfall the climate is on the whole mild, with no extremes of temperature; but a dry climate is one of extremes. A damp climate also causes people to feel keenly even slight changes of temperature. During the tropical wet season they feel cold even if the temperature is not really very low 65°–70° F.) and a temperature of 90–95° makes them feel very hot.

6. Effect of Large Sheets of Water.—As we should expect from our consideration of the effects of rain, the effect of seas and lakes on climate is to moderate it, that is, to keep the temperature of the land even. Near the equator the temperature on the coast seldom rises much above 95° F., whereas in the interior it may rise above 115°. Similarly in the cold season, the coast temperature rarely drops below 70°, whereas the interior sometimes has very cold nights (50° or less).

7. Effect of Trees and Vegetation.—Large forests increase the rainfall of an area, and the cutting down of forests has sometimes considerably reduced it. The leaves of trees and vegetation also protect the soil from the sun, and thus prevent it from drying up quickly. This keeps the land damp and so moderates the temperature.

8. Mountains and Valleys.—Mountains tend to increase the rainfall. They drive the winds high up into the sky where it is cold, and the cold makes the moisture in the winds condense and fall as rain. Mountains also shelter low lands from wind. Deep valleys are not usually healthy spots; they may be damp and misty. Winds coming down from high land are dry and cool and not often so violent as some ocean winds. So lands sheltered by mountains often have a bracing climate, one which makes people feel strong and active.

CLIMATE AND CHARACTER

Those who founded most of the ancient progressive civilizations both of the old and new worlds lived in tropical or sub-tropical countries. On the other hand, the founders of present-day civilization lived in the temperate climate of Europe and America. Yet many white people have tried to prove that their own climate was the only one to produce energetic, thinking, civilized people. One still hears the English weather praised and that of the tropics condemned, as if some tropical peoples were just at present less civilized than the white races *because of the climate*.

It is more reasonable to belive that *disease* is what had hindered their progress in civilization. If this be the case, we may reasonably hope that progress in tropical lands will be greater in the future than in the past. For though the tropics provide conditions very favourable to the growth of germs and disease-carrying insects, our knowledge of medicine and sanitation has of recent years made rapid advances. In the last 20 years large areas of the tropics have been cleared of malaria; tuberculosis and leprosy have become curable; and hardly any diseases remain as serious barriers to progress. If this knowledge can be intelligently applied by the people themselves, the conditions of their life may be fundamentally changed.

PERSONAL HEALTH

Chapter 24

BODY-HEAT AND CLOTHING

The body has an average temperature of 98·4° F.
This heat is obtained by the oxidation or " burning "
of our food which takes place within our bodies, and
from hot objects, such as the sun, fires and hot foods
and drinks. Heat is lost directly by the skin and by the
lungs when the body is surrounded by cold air and cold
objects, but mainly by *evaporation*. After getting wet
with perspiration, you feel cold as the perspiration
dries up. We have seen (page 101) that the skin itself
controls the amount of heat lost by evaporation by
regulating the flow of perspiration; to aid the skin in
this work we need clothing.

WHY CLOTHES ARE WORN

Clothes are used to keep the body warm in cold
weather and to shelter it from the sun in hot weather.
They protect the skin from injury and from rain, hail
and snow. But even where the climate makes clothes
unnecessary for health or comfort, they are still worn
for appearance. They also deal with the perspiration,
and with the circulation of air around the body.

Conductors of Heat.—Materials which allow heat to
pass through them easily are called *good conductors* of

heat. If we hold a piece of iron in a fire we find that the heat soon passes along the iron and burns our hand, iron being a good conductor. On the other hand materials like wool or flannelette, which will not let heat pass through them easily, are called *bad conductors*. Clothing which conducts heat badly is better than clothing made of good conductors. If the weather is hot, bad conductors keep the heat out; if cold, they keep the heat in.

Absorption of Perspiration.—In the tropics the body is usually damp, and often quite wet, with sweat. If this sweat is allowed to stay on the skin it is liable to cause a chill owing to its rapid evaporation, for, as we have seen, evaporation causes loss of heat. It is safer and more pleasant to let it evaporate slowly. So clothing material ought to be able to *absorb moisture*.

Reflection of Rays.—It is found that white clothing reflects the heat of the sun very effectively so that less heat passes through it to the body. On the other hand, black clothes absorb the heat and do not reflect it well. Hence in the tropics people should wear light coloured clothes in preference to dark ones. The fashion of wearing black suits on Sundays and special occasions is not a very good one, for, except on chilly days, they cause the body to be over-heated.

Circulation of Air.—Clothing in the tropics should thus be non-conducting, absorbent and light in colour. It should also be loose; if clothes are loose, and allow plenty of air to circulate about them, they will keep the body cool. In cold counties, clothing is made to retain air. Air being a bad conductor of heat, it acts like a blanket and keeps one warm. European men's clothing is meant to do this. Also, European suits are usually unwashable and therefore *not allowed to touch the skin*. This involves the wearing of washable underclothing, without which the suit soon begins to stink.

MATERIALS

The chief materials used for making clothes are:

1. Cotton.—This is the most widely used material for clothing in the tropics. It is made from the cotton plant and its fibres are like narrow twisted ribbons. It is

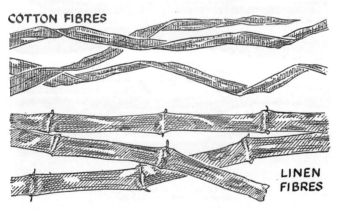

COTTON FIBRES

LINEN FIBRES

Fig. 69.—Cotton and Linen Fibres. (Highly magnified.)

inferior to wool as regards power of absorbing moisture, but is a fairly bad conductor of heat. It is cheap and strong, does not shrink much and washes well.

" *Flannelette* " is a cloth made from cotton which feels like wool. It is warm and absorbent but is dangerous for children as it easily catches fire. Non-inflammable flannelette is now made; it should be used for children's flannelette clothing.

Cotton is also made into " *cellular* " cloths which are

very suitable for wear in the tropics, as they permit the air to circulate freely in them and thus allow perspiration to dry up gradually.

2. Silk.—Silk is pleasant to wear. Its fibres are very smooth. It is a thread spun by the silk-worm and is a good material for clothes. It is a bad conductor of heat, and is quite strong when made into cloth. For

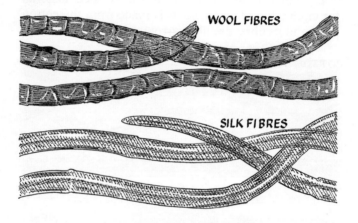

Fig. 70.—The Fibres of Wool and Silk seen under the Microscope. Note the small Scales.

the tropics it is very useful, but the damp atmosphere of certain parts is apt to cause it to perish quickly. Another disadvantage is its cost. Again, it is usually woven so as to prevent the breeze from cooling the body. Artificial silk and rayon have most of the qualities of real silk and are now widely used instead of it. So are nylon, orlon and other factory-made cloths.

3. Linen.—Linen is another vegetable product. Its fibres under the microscope have the appearance of sugar-cane. Linen is pleasant to wear, but not very absorbent. Flax from which it is made does not grow in the tropics, but linen is imported for its attractive appearance.

4. Wool.—This is most valuable in Europe as it is a bad conductor and retains moisture. Woollen cloth has within it many small holes or spaces which contain air and this again prevents heat from passing through the cloth. Wool has to be washed carefully. It contains a natural oil, and hot water with too much soap will wash this away. Hence only *warm water* should be used with *little soap*. Wool has the disadvantages of being rather expensive, of washing badly and shrinking, and of being rough to the skin. To overcome these, clothes are also made of wool mixed with other materials. It also retains heat in the body and causes overheating by preventing evaporation. It need only be considered in a book of tropical hygiene while European fashions are being copied in the tropics.

Waterproof Clothing.—In the wet season it is important to have some waterproof covering. This is usually in the form of a raincoat or a plastic "mackintosh". The disadvantage is that it prevents the perspiration from evaporating; so, while being protected from the wet outside, one becomes hot and wet inside the raincoat. It is useful for short errands; but on a bush journey, it is better to wrap your clothes in it, and let the rain wet your body. When the rain stops, or you reach shelter, your clothes are dry and ready for use.

Shoes and Sandals.—These are important articles of clothing and should be worn, especially in the wet season. Many diseases and sores are caused through the skin of the feet being punctured by stones, worms or jiggers. Boots and shoes should be of full size and give plenty of room for the toes.

Head Coverings.—These are used to protect the head from rain and sun and to shade the eyes from glare. Black hair is a natural protection from the sun, and curly hair encloses air which is a bad conductor of heat. In the heat of the day, however, extra protection is desirable. An ideal covering should reflect the sun's rays and provide for free ventilation between the head and the covering. It should also be light. These conditions are fulfilled by sun-helmets, straw hats, and light felt hats, the brims of which also shade the eyes; but not by the cloth cap, turban or fez.

AMOUNT OF CLOTHING REQUIRED

This varies according to the climate or season and the age or health of the person concerned.

Climate and Season.—In the tropics the amount of clothing required is small, its main duties being to look nice and protect the body from the sun's heat, and not to preserve bodily heat. In tropical coastal areas clothing will not change much in quantity throughout the year; but in the interior, where the temperature changes greatly with the seasons and even from day to night, care must be taken to increase the amount of clothing when necessary. The best guide is common sense. If you feel cold, wear more clothing whatever the time of year, and always be on guard against *sudden* drops in the temperature.

Age.—Except when running about, when it is cold children require clothing more than adults. Their skin is greater in area compared with their size than the skins of adults and therefore they lose heat more quickly. They should be clothed well. In the tropics naked children get bitten by flies and mosquitoes, they get cut, they get dirty and dusty, and germs of disease easily find their way into their bodies (see yaws, page 166).

Old people are less active and their bodies produce less heat. They need more clothing therefore than vigorous men.

Health.—A sick person, whose bodily functions are out of order, needs, as a rule, to wear more clothing. He needs warmth to recover from his disease, and extra clothing will save some of this body-heat. A sick man does not produce as much heat as a healthy one, and he is more likely to catch a chill. Even during fevers warm clothing is required to prevent a chill.

VALUE OF SUNLIGHT

When tropical diseases were little understood, the sun was blamed for much ill-health, and sunstroke was much talked about. But the sun is not the cause of much sickness, except sunburn among white-skinned people whose skin may blister by exposure to bright sun unless protected by clothing or sun-tan oil. *Heat exhaustion* is a kind of fainting coming on after exertion in the heat. With salty drinks and cool air and cold water sponging people soon recover. *Heat Stroke* results when sweating fails after long walking or work in great heat. There is fever, dry hot skin and coma. People may die if not quickly cooled.

The sun has great health-giving properties. It prevents some kinds of ringworm, and helps in the formation of vitamins. Working in the sun, and even sun-bathing, are good so long as sunburn and heat-stroke are avoided.

Chapter 25

CARE OF THE PERSON

EXERCISE

It is important at all periods of life to take sufficient exercise. Sometimes this exercise is provided in our daily work. A blacksmith is continually exercising his muscles. If, however, our work does not include a good amount of bodily activity, we must take care to get it daily in some other way. Children especially need exercise. Hence games and sports are a necessary part of a child's life and should be encouraged. But there is such a thing as *over-exercise*. Actually nature always warns us when a wise limit has been reached: we feel tired, and stop the game.

Effect of Exercise on the Body.

1. The muscles are enlarged and strengthened.
2. The heart becomes stronger and beats more rapidly, causing an increased flow of blood to every part of the body.
3. The lungs are increased in size, and this means more efficient purification of the blood.
4. The skin perspires freely, thus getting rid of impurities in the blood.
5. The nerves are strengthened owing to the increased blood supply.

6. The excretory organs (bowels and kidneys) are made to act more efficiently.

7. The digestion is improved and the appetite made keener.

Training.—Sometimes, through necessity or fool-hardiness, a man makes his body do an unusual amount of work without due training for it. This is bad and may result in serious trouble. Exercise to be beneficial must be taken regularly. If this is done the body will by degrees be able to increase the amount it can do. A boy who attempts to run a mile quickly without previous practice will not only fail but will also be in danger of injuring his heart. If he first takes short runs and gradually increases the distance, he will, after a month or two, be able to run a fast mile and will strengthen his body in so doing. This is called being in training.

Although exercise mainly concerns the body, its effects are also seen upon the mind. A person who takes little exercise is apt to be slow in mind as well as in body. Although the brain requires its own special kind of activity such as reading and study, yet it also needs to be nourished with good blood; and this can only be produced by a healthy and active body. Thus a healthy mind is usually found in a healthy body. In some cases general ill-health results simply from lack of exercise.

Swimming.—This is one of the best forms of exercise. Every school should try to organize it. If the sea, or fast-flowing rivers, or places where crocodiles or sharks may be a danger, are used for school swims, strict precautions must be taken to prevent accidents. For instance, no-one should swim alone; a teacher in swimming costume must watch from the shore or from a boat. If there are too many for the teacher in charge to count all the time, then everyone should have a swimming-mate who will shout to the teacher if his mate cannot be seen. It must be a strict rule that no-one should pretend to be in danger. Sea-snakes bite and some jelly-fish are poisonous. If the water is unclean epidemics may be spread by it, but this is rare. It has been known for cholera to be caught from river water. No such danger comes from sea bathing.

Every school should aim to have a swimming pool. Often part of a stream can be deepened and kept clear. If not, a pool may have to be dug, lined with cement and filled from the water pipes. Two things are needed to make such a pool healthy: a filter and treatment machine to deal with germs in the water; and showers, so that everyone can bath with soap before entering the pool. Even with all these precautions, it is common to find an increase of fungus trouble on the feet when people are using swimming pools. A foot bath with disinfectant between the showers and the pool helps to guard against this. Girls must not swim when they are having a monthly period.

Sport.—All boys and girls, unless certified by a doctor as physically unfit, ought to play regular games of some kind. Games ought to provide for the exercise of all parts of the body and not merely the legs. Most games exercise only one set of muscles. Thus *football* exercises mainly the legs, and other games which bring different muscles into use ought to be played as well.

Rules.—We may summarize rules concerning exercise as follows:

1. It should be taken regularly.

2. It should not be violent or last too long.

3. It should, if possible, be taken in the open air.

4. It should exercise all parts of the body. Tennis, swimming, gymnastics and walking are excellent in this respect.

5. It should not be taken soon after a meal or when tired.

6. Care should be taken after exercise to avoid a chill. For this reason special clothing should be worn which can be completely changed after the exercise.

REST

Rest is as necessary to health as exercise. As the muscles and organs of the body do their work they wear out, that is, they lose part of their substance. They need building up. Further, a well-exercised muscle always has to become bigger than it was before. It is during rest that this takes place. Even those organs, like the heart and the lungs, which seem never to rest, have their regular periods of repose. The heart rests more than half its time.

Sleep is the only perfect form of rest, and it is most important for health that sleep should be regular and sufficient.

Rules for Sleep.—No definite rule can be given as to the number of hours one ought to sleep, as the amount varies according to age, sex, temperament and work. Children require a lot of sleep and should go to bed early, say at 7 p.m., and sleep till morning. Boys and girls ought to retire not later than 9 or 9.30 p.m. Adults vary in the amount of sleep they require but usually seven to nine hours are necessary.

A habit of going to bed after 11 p.m. may be kept up by some, but with most people it will have bad effects. It is a law of nature that night should not be turned into day, and the hours between 10 p.m. and 5 a.m. are those during which sleep is most beneficial.

Women require more sleep than men as they get more easily fatigued with work. Students should rarely " burn the midnight oil "; their best work is done when the brain is fresh.

General Rules for Sleep may be summarized as follows—

1. Children should have plenty of sleep at night and also rest during the day.

2. Boys and girls should go to bed about 9.30 p.m., and adults not later than 11 p.m.

3. Brain workers and women require more sleep than do manual labourers and men.

4. A short rest after lunch is beneficial (see page 59).

5. The bedroom should be clean and airy.

6. Food should not be taken immediately before going to bed for the night.

7. The body should be kept warm during sleep.

Weekly Rest Day.—A change of occupation for one day in seven is in itself a health-giving practice. If this day is devoted to getting strength from the Creator of our bodies and minds so as to keep them doing good work, it is still better.

REGULAR HABITS

Most people understand the importance of the formation of good habits of conduct, but few realize how important it is to have regular habits with regard to such things as eating, drinking and sleeping. What does " habit " mean? The oftener we do anything the easier it is for us to do it again, and this continues until we can do some things without thinking about them at all. A person who goes to bed regularly at 10 p.m. will find his body ready for sleep at that hour and will have no desire to sit up later. Regular habits, therefore, are an aid to good health, and they should be carefully cultivated in respect of—

1. Sleep.—The brain will be ready for sleep at the usual hour if this is regularly kept.

2. Meal Times.—We saw in our study of constipation (see page 95) that regular meals were an aid against this trouble. The stomach requires regular hours of work and rest, and if we eat too often and at irregular times the stomach will miss this rest and may soon be so out of order that constipation, indigestion and other ills may follow. With meals at regular times the organs of digestion will be ready for their work at the same hours every day and things will go smoothly.

3. Opening the Bowels.—This, too, should be regular. One of the chief ways of avoiding constipation is to find time at a certain hour every day to clear the bowels; if this is regularly kept up the habit will soon be formed.

4. Cleanliness.—Mention has already been made of the care of the teeth (see page 84). The habit of cleaning them after breakfast and supper should be formed, in childhood if possible. It is obvious that good habits of washing, bathing and the care of the hair, nails and ears are a great help too.

BATHING

The Daily Bath.—First, decide which is the most convenient time for bathing. Some prefer the early morning, immediately on rising, but others prefer an evening bath. Having fixed the time, keep to it regularly, and it will prove a valuable help in the preservation of health. A bath is not necessary, a bucket or a shower is as good.

Washing the Hands.—Hands should be washed with soap and water several times a day, and the habit should be formed of always washing before eating.

THE HAIR

The hair should be regularly washed, brushed and combed. This is even more necessary for curly than for straight hair as curly hair retains dust and insects very easily. It is unwise, however, to use soap, especially coarse soap, too often on the hair.

THE NAILS

The nails should be kept short as dirt is easily collected under them. They should be cut with a pair of scissors or filed, and not bitten. A brush should be used to scrub them as it is important that they should be kept quite clean.

THE EYES

The greatest care ought to be taken of the eyes as they are precious, and any defect or irritation ought to be seen to at once by a qualified doctor. There is, however, nothing to be gained from eye drops and lotions if the eyes are not actually sick.

Defective Sight.—A person shows that his eyes are not normal by one or more of the following signs, and he ought to have them attended to at once.

1. He holds his book near his face or far away.

2. He holds his head sideways or shuts one eye in order to see clearly.

3. He blinks frequently or complains of the glare.

4. He has frequent headaches.

5. He reads badly from charts or the blackboard even though he can read well from books.

Often these troubles can be put right by early attention. Even the discovery that one eye sees more clearly than the other should be enough to make the person go to a doctor.

EYE TROUBLES

Various diseases of the eyes are common in hot countries and some of these are very infectious. The subject of eye diseases can only be touched on here, but one or two simple precautions and remedies may be mentioned.

Prevention.—Handkerchiefs, towels and pillows are common ways in which germs go from a bad eye of one person to the good eye of someone else. Persons suffering from eye trouble often want to rub their eyes with their fingers or handkerchief. Anyone suffering from a sore eye should wash his hands after touching it. His towels, handkerchiefs and pillow should be kept apart from other people's, and all cotton-wool and rags used to wash the eye should afterwards be burned.

" Pink Eye ".—Sometimes you see a child with very sore-looking eyes. They are red and a thin slimy discharge comes out of them. This may be due to the germs of gonorrhœa or other microbes. The discharge is contagious and if it gets into another person's eyes it will cause the disease; it must be attended to by a *qualified doctor*.

Treatment.—Dissolve a teaspoonful of boric acid in

P

a pint of water which has been boiled, and bathe the eye with this lotion twice a day. Add a little hot water to the lotion before use. The eye may be washed out by means of a teapot if a proper irrigator is not available. Afterwards anoint the lids with some albucid or penicillin ointment, vaseline or castor oil. Ask the doctor for exact orders. The eye must be treated with the proper medicine, not bush medicines.

Never put a pad over an eye which is discharging. If the patient fears the light let him wear a shade and stay in a quiet light; do not keep him in the dark.

Eye Ulcers.—If a person cannot stand the light and complains of a pricking sensation in the eye, it is possible that he may be suffering from an ulcer in the eye. There may be redness as well. In this case it is always safe to wash the eye with boric lotion. But all cases of eye trouble must go to a doctor. An eye which merely itches for a few weeks, and gets slightly red, may have a serious disease: *trachoma*, for instance, which is infectious and a common cause of blindness, starts in this mild fashion.

THE EARS

These very delicate and important organs should be looked after. They should be washed daily with soap and water in order to clear away dust which may sometimes have gathered there.

Earache is a warning that there is something wrong with the ear. On no account should anything be put into the ear just to stop the irritation. Earache may be due to a simple cold with slight inflammation of the ear. On the other hand it may be the result of far more serious trouble, and if earache continues more than a day or so, a doctor should be seen and the ear examined.

Discharge from the Ear.—This is a serious symptom and it is of great importance that it should be medically treated at once. If pus comes out, it may have punctured the drum of the ear; if not attended to, the hearing may be affected permanently. There is also a grave danger lest the pus may discharge *inside* the head and cause death. Anyone with a discharge from the ear ought to see a doctor at once.

Wax protects the ear-drum from insects and should not be removed; any excess may be removed with the little finger. If the ear is blocked with wax, the doctor may have to wash it out. Some people's ears allow water to get in and this may cause the wax to swell. Anyone to whom this has happened should put cotton-wool in the ears before going for a swim.

Chapter 26

ACCIDENTS

There are occasions when a little knowledge of " first aid " will enable people to render very useful service. At any time an accident may take place in which some immediate treatment of the patient is required. It must, however, be distinctly understood in what follows that the treatment is only of an emergency kind, and in all cases of serious accident a doctor should be informed. It is important for the doctor that the messenger should be able to state clearly the nature of the accident.

WOUNDS AND CUTS

These are common, and immediate attention is required. There are three kinds of bleeding according as the blood comes from the capillaries, arteries or veins.

Ordinary Cuts and Scratches are usually accompanied by capillary bleeding. This, the least serious kind of bleeding, is the ooze from wounds and grazes. They should all be treated to prevent germs from developing in them. Acriflavine is better for this than iodine, and a firm bandage over this dressing usually stops the bleeding.

If it does not stop on being tightly bandaged, it is probably arterial bleeding. This is bright red and may have been seen spurting with each heart-beat from one point in the wound. Blood from veins is darker red and flows out steadily.

To stop Serious Bleeding.—The rule is, " press on the bleeding spot "—the point in the wound from which most blood is coming. Press here, using both thumbs if necessary, and do not let go. If the dressing has been put on, press over it.

While waiting for the doctor, put a pad and very tight bandage on the wound. If blood is then seen soaking rapidly into the dressing, press on this with both thumbs again. Such pressure on the wound very rarely fails to stop the bleeding. Special methods for stopping it in various parts of the body should be learned from First Aid Manuals.

Varicose Veins.—These are enlarged veins, most frequently of the legs. If they burst or are cut, a great deal of blood flows. In such a case act as follows:

(1) Let the patient lie down and raise the wounded leg.

(2) Bind a pad over the bleeding spot.

Note.—In all cases of severe bleeding the first thing is to stop the flow of blood. Do not be anxious if the patient faints, as fainting means that the blood is circulating less rapidly and this helps to stop the flow. Never give stimulants, but see that the patient's clothing is loose and that he has plenty of fresh air.

A severe wound will often clean itself by bleeding, but when the bleeding has been stopped the wound should be well washed, so that no dirt, sand or grit remains in it. This should be done with acriflavine solution; every home and school should have some. The skin around the wound must be cleaned.

Nose Bleeding.—This is common. To treat it—

1. Make the patient sit on a chair with his head thrown *backwards.*

2. Apply cold water to the forehead and nose, or, better still, ice may be applied, if available.

3. Loosen the clothing round the chest and throat, and let the patient sit in a current of air. Fan him if necessary to provide this.

4. Nearly all nose bleeding is from just within the nostril, on the side near the middle of the nose. It can be stopped by gently squeezing the whole nose for a few minutes, followed by gentle pressure on the side that was bleeding. It is often prevented by cutting the patient's nails short so that he does not pick his nose.

Bleeding from the Tongue.—Let the patient stuff the end of a clean towel into his mouth, or some cotton-wool, and press hard on the tongue. If the cut is deep, press the sides of the wound with the fingers until bleeding stops.

Blood spitting.—This is usually from an injured or diseased lung and the blood is frothy in appearance. Let the patient lie down with his head to one side. Allow plenty of fresh air. Consult a doctor, for the patient may have tuberculosis.

FRACTURES

When a bone is broken it is said to be fractured. There are two main kinds of fractures, Simple and Compound. Simple fracture involves only the bone. The skin is not broken, and great care should be taken to see that it does not become so. Compound fracture is one where the skin over the bone is also broken. This is very much more serious because germs may pass into the bone through the wound.

Signs of Fracture.—1. The part is painful and swollen and has lost the power of movement.

2. The shape of the injured part may look wrong, and a limb is usually shortened; the broken arm or leg is shorter than the other.

3. The broken end of the bone can sometimes be seen or felt under the skin.

Treatment.—Fractures are a doctor's job. All fractures with a wound near by, however small, must be taken to hospital. All other cases in which a bone is broken, or where the first aid man is in doubt whether it is broken, should also be taken to the doctor. However, if a limb is fractured or too swollen or painful to move, it must be given first aid: that is, fix the bones so as to keep them still. This prevents the sharp end of the bone from piercing the skin or cutting an artery or vein while on the way to the doctor.

If the skin is broken the wound must be washed

with acriflavine solution. A pad soaked in this solution should then be placed upon it to prevent the entry of dust. If the wound is bleeding much, the *first* thing to do is to *stop the bleeding*.

Splints.—These are pieces of wood or some other rigid material which are tied firmly to the broken limb to keep it still. They may be made from any rigid article as a rolled-up newspaper or exercise

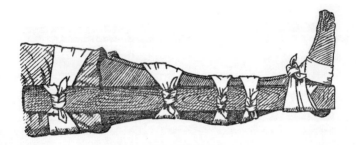

Fig. 71.—Splinting for Broken Shin-Bone.

book, an umbrella or walking-stick. Where it touches the limb the splint should be padded so that it will not hurt the patient. The pad may be made of any soft material—a folded shirt or towel, a bunch of grass, pieces of paper, or rags. When one leg is broken below the knee, tying it to the good leg is a good way to splint it.

Rules.—We may summarize the first aid treatment of fractures as follows:

1. Before attempting to move the patient fix the broken limb in splints. However great the temptation may be to carry him to a more convenient spot the

splinting must be done first, otherwise serious injury may result. Let the patient lie just where he is, even in the middle of a crowded street.

To keep both broken ends still, fix the joint above and the joint below. The splint must therefore extend beyond the upper and lower joints. In the case of a leg, the other leg may be used as a splint, and both the ankle (the joint below) and the knee (the joint above) must be fixed.

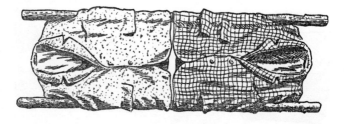

Fig. 72.—An Emergency Stretcher.

2. After splinting, it is good to bathe the injured part in cold water. If there is a wound, it must be carefully washed as explained above.

3. Keep the patient warm. After the shock of an accident the patient may faint. The face gets pale and the skin cold. Place clothing over him, and if he is conscious give him a hot drink.

4. Removal. If this is necessary, remember the patient must be carried as gently as possible, to save him pain and injury. A *stretcher* may be made in several ways. Any large flat article can be used, like a door or shutter taken off its hinges, or a sheet of corrugated iron. Two bamboos passed through the inverted sleeves of coats or through two sacks make an

emergency stretcher. If the patient is removed in a car or rickshaw, it should travel slowly. Do everything possible for the comfort of the patient.

5. If a thigh or leg is broken and you are sure that an ambulance will come, wait for it. The ambulance team ought to have a special splint called a Thomas splint as well as a good stretcher.

DISLOCATIONS

If bones slip away from each other at a joint, this is called a dislocation. The change of shape, which is also seen in fractures, here occurs at a joint, and is nearly always obvious. The patient cannot use the limb.

Dislocated bones are mostly very difficult to replace properly. It is a doctor's job. The doctor will be able to do it better if the joint has first been treated for the sprain which always accompanies dislocation. So the first aid treatment is given below.

SPRAINS

These occur when a joint is violently twisted, wrenched or over-exercised. Any joint may be thus sprained, the most common being the wrist and ankle. The swelling is due to extra joint fluid, commonly called " water "; a sprained knee is called " water on the knee ".

Signs.—(1) Pain and swelling, usually coming on gradually in the case of sprains. (2) Loss of power.

Treatment.—(1) Bind the joint firmly with a bandage. (2) Pour cold water over the bandage and keep it cold and wet. Better still, the joint may be put under a running tap. (3) Next day, apply *hot* fomentations. (4) Rest the joint by putting it in a splint or sling.

A sprained joint may take a long time to recover; it ought not to be used until recovery is complete.

BRUISES

A bruise results from a heavy blow or a fall. The skin swells and becomes discoloured because blood from the broken capillaries is loose in the tissues. Very bad bruises must be treated as for sprains; if the patient cannot use the bruised part, treat it as if it were a fracture.

Rather similar swellings result from tearing muscles or ligaments; and as the treatment is the same, they are here dealt with together.

BURNS

Burns are extremely painful and often serious. A big area slightly burnt is more dangerous than a deeper small burn. Scalds are produced by hot water or steam touching the skin. The treatment is the same as for for burns, as follows—

1. Treat for Shock.—A severe burn or scald always causes shock to the system and there is danger of the patient fainting under it. Cover him up lightly. If he is conscious give him a little warm sweet tea to drink.

2. Cover the Area of the Burn so as to exclude air from it. To do this remove the patient's clothes very carefully so as not to tear the skin. If the burn is on a limb it should be placed in a warm bath. Cover small burns with oil spread on strips of clean linen or lint. The oil most used for this purpose, Liquid Paraffin, is a useful oil to keep handy. Failing this other oils may be used, such as *olive oil*, *cod-liver oil*, *vaseline* or *palm oil*. Then cover with cotton wool to exclude air, and bandage.

But if the burn is so serious that a doctor must see it, oil must not be used, as it spoils the doctor's treatment. Instead of oil, bathe the part in a warm solution of baking soda (sodium bicarbonate); or break an egg over it; or sprinkle flour or baking soda on it. The burn may first be painted with warm weak picric acid or acriflavine solution to kill germs.

The above, however, are makeshift methods. The proper treatment is triple dye jelly. This is sold in tubes, and only needs squeezing out and spreading on the burn. Deep or large burns should be taken to the doctor immediately after this first aid.

3. Do not open blisters.—A blister is the perfect dressing for a burn. Broken blisters, however, will be cut away by the doctor or nurse.

Clothes on Fire.—If anyone's clothes catch fire, often the first thing he does is to run about wild with fear. This naturally causes the flames to burn more fiercely and he may burn to death. Anyone may save life by acting as follows:

1. Make the person lie on the ground, by force if necessary, burning part uppermost if possible.

2. Put out the flames by wrapping cloth round him tightly. A table-cloth, curtain, sleeping cloth, carpet or mat, or one's own clothes, may be used for this purpose. If water is available it should be dashed on the burning clothes, but do not wait for this to be brought.

Many a person whose clothes have caught fire has saved his life by wrapping himself in some material or rolling about on the ground. The rolling itself, without a cloth, may put out the flames. In treating the burns, great care must be taken in removing the clothes. It is better to leave burnt pieces on the skin than to tear the blisters open.

DROWNING

There are several methods by which breathing can be restored to a person apparently drowned. The great thing is to commence work *at once* without wasting time, as every moment is precious. Schäfer's Method was formerly much used if there were no broken ribs—

(1) Without delay clear the patient's nose and mouth of any weeds or false teeth and pull the tongue forward. (2) Loosen the clothing about the neck and waist, and then commence artificial respiration. (3) While doing this, send someone for a doctor. (4) Other messengers should go to get blankets, hot drinks, dry clothes, and if possible an ambulance or other transport.

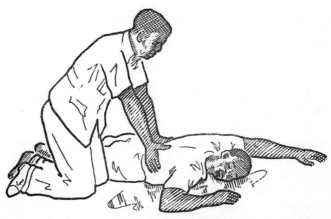

Fig. 73.—Schäfer's Method.

(*a*) Place the patient face downwards on the ground with the head sideways, and his arms above his head. (*b*) Pick him up by the hips and hold him head downwards while you count five; this will let water out of his air passages. (*c*) Kneel beside the patient and place your thumbs in the small of his back and fingers grasping his ribs. (*d*) Press downwards steadily. This will expel air. (*e*) Relax the pressure without moving your hands from his back. This allows air to flow into the lungs. Keep up these two movements by rocking your body *regularly* at the rate of about ten times a minute. Artificial respiration may have to be kept up a long time before breathing is restored. Cases have been known to come to life after several hours. Keep it up even in the ambulance. Do not let anyone stop you.

A simpler and more effective method is to inflate the patient's lungs by blowing them up through his nose. Place a handkerchief over his closed mouth and nose, hold the jaw up and the head back. Then put your wide open mouth over his nose and, through the handkerchief, blow out all your breath into him making his chest expand. Stop, let the air escape and repeat every five seconds. He may soon start a jerky shallow gasp of his own, but go on till he breathes properly.

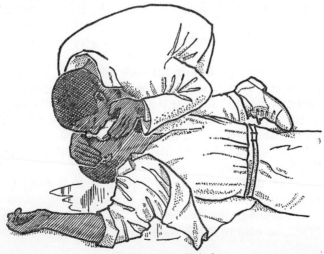

Fig. 74.—Inflation Method

After-treatment.—While doing all this, get someone (1) to remove the wet clothing and cover the patient with blankets, (2) to rub his limbs in a direction towards the heart. Afterwards get him taken to a house and put into bed and kept warm; see that he gets hot drinks.

CHOKING

If a person is choking through swallowing something like a fish-bone, or coin, he begins to go black in the face and gets very much alarmed. Prompt action is necessary and you must not lose your head. (1) Put your forefinger down his throat as far as you can and try to hook the thing out. Two or three attempts may have to be made but it is essential to remove it. (2) Thump his back while you bend the head forward or hold him up by the hips or feet, head downwards. (3) In extreme cases, artificial respiration may be necessary after the object has been removed.

FAINTING, SHOCK, COLLAPSE, STROKES, FITS

Fainting is fairly common in crowds. It is also called loss of consciousness, or shock, or collapse. It may be due to several causes, but there are *general rules* which may be applied in all cases.

1. Place the patient on his back and watch his face. If the face is pale let his head lie low so that blood may run into it. See that the neck is not bent in such a way as to make breathing difficult. If the face is flushed and dark let the head be raised.

2. Loosen all clothing about the neck and waist so that breathing may be easy.

3. Let there be plenty of fresh air. It is specially necessary to see to this if there is a crowd.

4. Smelling salts or a burning feather in front of the nose may help to revive the patient.

5. Place the patient in a cool spot, lay him down and rub his limbs.

6. Do not give any liquid to drink until patient has regained consciousness. Then give hot tea or coffee.

Epileptic Fits.—*Signs.* (1) The patient sometimes shows the approach of a fit in various ways. This would only be noticed by one who knew that the patient was liable to these fits and who was on the alert. (2) The patient becomes pale, utters a curious cry and falls down. (3) Convulsions occur; this means that the patient throws his arms and legs about. He may foam at the mouth, and the face muscles work. Epileptics usually pass urine during the fit. (4) It is followed by a period of quiet, after which the patient recovers consciousness and, except for a dazed look, appears well again.

Treatment.—Take care that the patient does not injure himself by knocking his head on the ground or biting his tongue during the convulsions. To prevent this, place a cork or pencil between his teeth, put a cushion of some kind under his head and hold him *gently* to prevent his movements from hurting him. Put a handkerchief or the corner of a cloth in his hands to prevent his nails from digging into them.

When the fit is over let the patient rest and then let him go about his business. Do not make a fuss over him but watch to see if the fit occurs again. Epilepsy should be treated by a doctor; it can sometimes be cured.

Heatstroke (including sunstroke) comes on suddenly. The face of the patient is flushed and he has a high temperature—104–110° F. He sometimes becomes very excited and even delirious and this is succeeded by collapse and unconsciousness.

Treatment.—The patient should be put in a cool place, his clothes removed, covered with a sheet or towel wrung out of cold water, and fanned to cool him down by evaporation. Do not continue this after his temperature has been reduced to 100°.

It is possible that the patient may sink into a state of collapse after his temperature has come down, so you must be prepared to treat for collapse in the way already described. Blankets must be wrapped round him to keep him warm, and hot sweet tea given. He must see a doctor, for it is possible that it is malaria, and this needs urgent treatment. If a doctor cannot see him the same day, give him malaria treatment (p. 140).

POISONS

The study of poisons is a very complicated one and all we can do is just to mention some of the general facts about them.

Signs of Poisoning.—Poisoning may be suspected—

1. If a healthy man is suddenly seized with internal pains. (Though certain diseases start in this way also.)

2. If several people who have eaten the same food together, especially tinned foods or fish, experience the same symptoms. This is called food poisoning.

General Treatment.

1. Send for a doctor at once.

2. In all cases—*except where the patient's lips and mouth are stained by the poison*—try to make him vomit (see below). Medicines to cause vomiting are called emetics.

3. Give castor oil to clear out the bowel—two table-spoonfuls for an adult.

4. Let the patient take some milk, or eggs beaten

up in milk, or oil. Suitable oils are olive oil, palm oil, or coconut oil.

To cause Vomiting.—Either (1) Put your finger down the patient's throat; or (2) Give him salt water to drink—a tablespoonful of salt in a cup of warm water is a useful emetic; or (3) Let him drink some warm water mixed with mustard—a dessertspoonful of mustard in a large cupful of water.

Stains about the mouth show the presence of strong acids or alkalies. Never give an emetic in these cases because the poison vomited up will do further damage.

When the Poison is Known.—If the poison is known, special treatment can be given by a doctor which will undo the effects of the poison. The medicine given is called the " antidote ".

Narcotics.—These produce a desire to sleep. Many medicines, contain these poisons, and if taken in excess may produce bad results. Opium, Indian hemp, and sometimes alcohol, are narcotics.

Treatment:
1. Make the patient vomit.
2. Give him strong coffee to drink.
3. Prevent him from sleeping by forcing him to walk about and slapping him with the hand.

Note: Many people have the habit of taking patent medicines as soon as they feel unwell. This is a bad habit. Medicines should only be taken on the advice of a responsible person.

HOME MEDICINE CUPBOARD

Some medicines are useful for small sicknesses, to prevent them from becoming big ones. You should have a locked cupboard or a box in your home with

Q

small quantities of aspirin (in 5-grain tablets), Epsom salts, bicarbonate of soda, malaria tablets, liquid paraffin and castor oil.

On a different shelf keep some medicines to kill germs, such as potassium permanganate, Dettol, acriflavine solution and triple dye jelly for burns or cuts, and boric acid powder. It is good to keep with these medicines some clean white cloth for dressings, some strips of cloth of any colour for bandages, some cotton wool and a few safety pins.

Chapter 27

STATE HEALTH SERVICES

There is in nearly all tropical countries a Government Medical Department or perhaps a Ministry of Health. There may also be Mission Medical services or other voluntary or commercial medical activities, but the Government must look upon the welfare of its people as a matter of national concern and not merely a personal or family matter. That is why welfare states are bringing in some sort of National Health Service for the protection of the people's health and to give free treatment to those who require it, though private doctors, nurses and others are still allowed to practise and charge fees.

The Curative Services are based on Hospitals, Dispensaries and Clinics where sick people can be treated, though where there are enough family doctors many people can be treated in their own homes, and this is much better when it can be done safely. A big town will have a large General Hospital where many doctors and specialists work together. There will be smaller regional and district hospitals, each surrounded by a number of rural dispensaries and clinics.

In order to train all the doctors and nurses and other helpers there must be a University Hospital where specialists from other countries can help if need be, and where research can be carried on to discover more about illness and its treatment.

Preventive Services are under the care of Medical Officers of Health who have offices for records and publicity work. They are helped by Health Inspectors, Midwives, Community nurses etc., often working with doctors or medical assistants in Health Centres. Then there must be Central Pharmacies for medicines and the hospital supplies, and ambulances for the transport of the sick, laboratories and X-ray centres.

The rural areas have to be served by mobile units whose duty is to tackle endemic diseases like yaws and leprosy and sleeping sickness and organize treatment centres or special settlements, like the famous leper colonies which are doing so much good.

Infectious Diseases Hospitals may also be needed and there is a growing need for Mental Hospitals where those who are mentally sick can be cared for and often cured. Last but not least in importance is the School Medical Service which is meant to watch over the health of the children.

Dental Services are lagging behind the others, but they are badly needed both for preventive and curative work.

HOUSING CONDITIONS

As we have seen, these have a lot to do with health, for overcrowding in slums favours the spread of the air-borne and the contact diseases. Regulations are laid down about the kind of building which is permitted in any given area, and people should not be allowed to build anyhow and anywhere. Health Inspectors help to see that the regulations about drains and sewers, latrines and water supplies are observed. They also have to inspect slaughter houses and prevent bad meat from being sold, and to see that markets are kept clean and that restaurants and eating houses observe the sanitary laws.

STATISTICS

Every now and then the Government carries out a *Census*, which means a counting of the number of people living in various districts with their sex, age and occupation and many other facts about their lives. It is very important for the Health Department to have this information in order to plan properly for the medical needs of the population. But ordinary statistics, as these figures are called, are not enough. We need to know not only how many people are being born each year, but how many of these survive and grow up. We also want to know what are the main diseases from which people die or from which they suffer. These figures are called *Vital Statistics*—birth rate, death rate, infant mortality rate, sickness (or morbidity) rate, etc. These figures may vary in different parts of the country, or among different tribes or different classes of workers. If they are found to be very high the reason must be looked for in poor diet, insanitary conditions or the presence of too many insect hosts of disease.

CENTRAL AND LOCAL GOVERNMENT

In order to run the health services the Central Ministry of Health has to work closely with the Local

Government agencies, whether they be Sultans, Chiefs or Headmen, or elected members of Councils. Every town wants to have its own hospital and every large village its own dispensary, but an overall plan must decide when and where these can be provided. It depends on the number of doctors and nurses available and on the money which can be spent, most of which must come from the taxes we pay. Sometimes a local community can club together and build a health centre or a dispensary and help to pay the salary of the workers or to buy medicines. There will always be room for self-help, however advanced our welfare state has got.

NOTIFICATION

There is a list of the diseases which must be notified to the Medical Officer of Health, and doctors are made responsible for doing this. Cases must not be hidden for fear of serious epidemics breaking out. Most people now know that there are many wonderful medicines for curing most diseases so that they are becoming more willing to seek help. It is so important that any case of what appears to be serious illness should have medical help as early as possible, and not wait till too late, either from fear or from trying all sorts of old fashioned medicines. There are many wicked people about who try to sell useless medicines for which they claim wonderful cures, and many advertisements which are false and deceive those who know no better.

YOU AND THE HEALTH SERVICE

Before you leave school, give a thought about a job in the health service. There are many ways in which you could make a good and useful career in it.

Ask your teacher, doctor or Health Inspector.

QUESTIONS FOR HOMEWORK
AND REVISION

The pupil is recommended to draw diagrams wherever possible to illustrate his answers.

CHAPTER 1

1. Define the words " Sanitation " and " Hygiene " so as to show the difference between them.
2. What do all living things need? What must they be able to do in order to survive?
3. How can the body be aided in its fight against disease?
4. Why is the study of hygiene especially important in tropical countries?
5. What is physiology? Mention five of the systems of which the body consists.
6. Into what main groups are the causes of disease divided? How are we defended against them?

CHAPTER 2

1. Give the approximate composition of the air, and say what you know of its constituents.
2. Why is breathing like burning?
3. Why does not the air become full of carbon dioxide through people breathing and things burning?
4. How does the composition of expired air differ from that of ordinary air?
5. Give some of the evil effects of overcrowding.
6. Write a short account of the cause, spread and prevention of tuberculosis.

CHAPTER 3

1. What is meant by ventilation? Why is it necessary?
2. Explain the terms " Artificial " and " Natural " ventilation. What properties of air are used in natural ventilation?
3. What methods of artificial ventilation are used? Where are they chiefly to be seen?

4. What objections are there to the ventilation of rooms at night by means of open doors and windows? How may they be overcome?
5. Explain how modern houses can be ventilated and draw diagrams of any apparatus used.
6. (a) How would you test for the presence of Carbon Dioxide?
   (b) How can you prove that hot air has less weight than cold air?

CHAPTER 4

1. What are the qualities of water which is good for drinking?
2. Write a list of the sources of water putting them under the heads " Good ", " Suspicious ", " Dangerous ".
3. Draw a diagram showing how a spring may be formed. What do you know about spring water?
4. Distinguish between " Surface " and " Deep " wells. Draw diagrams to illustrate your answers.
5. If your yard has a shallow well, what precautions will you take to keep the water good?
6. Why are rivers dangerous to drink from?
7. What are common impurities in water and what are their effects on one who drinks them?
8. Define the terms " Hard " and " Soft " water. What are the disadvantages of hard water? Has it any advantages?
9. How can hard water be softened?
10. If the water in a village is obviously dirty what would you do before drinking it?
11. Give the common means of purifying water and describe fully how to make a simple filter.

CHAPTER 5

(a)

1. What are the uses of food?
2. Make a table to show the different main groups of food.
3. Why does the body need water?
4. Give the names of some common proteins and say what you know of them.
5. Why are fats and oils required by the body? What foods contain them?
6. What foods give us sugars? Which ones give starches? What can you say about starch as a food?
7. Why are fruits good to eat?

(b)

1. Which is the better food, beef or pork? Give your reasons.
2. Say what you know of fish as a food.
3. What is the value of milk as a food? How can we keep it free from germs?
4. What is (a) Cream, (b) Cheese, (c) Butter?
   How are they produced?
5. Give the composition of eggs. How can they be preserved?

(c)

1. What are the chief cereal foods? Write a short account of any two of them, and two other carbohydrate foods.
2. How is bread made? What is the special value of brown bread?
3. Give the various classes of vegetable foods. Why are green vegetables good for food?
4. Name some kinds of bean. Why are they able to take the place of meat in our diet?
5. Give the advantages and disadvantages of tinned foods.

CHAPTER 6

1. Give the constituents of tea. What is the effect of tea upon the body?
2. How should tea be made? What are the disadvantages of strong tea?
3. What are the special characteristics of coffee? Compare it with tea.
4. How should coffee be made?
5. " Cocoa is more of a food than a beverage." Explain this statement.
6. Distinguish between beers, wines and spirits as regards their manufacture and percentage of alcohol.
7. What are the effects of alcohol on the body?

CHAPTER 7

1. What are the advantages of a mixed diet? Give a few combinations of foods which provide a suitable meal.
2. Give the effects of (a) Under-feeding, (b) Over-feeding.
3. Give some rules concerning meals.
4. Why should food be cooked? Give some of the effects of good cooking on food.

5. Describe the following methods of cooking meat:
   Baking, Boiling, Stewing. What are their special effects on meat?
6. Why should a kitchen be kept clean? Describe a home-made meat safe.

CHAPTER 8

1. Why should we breathe through the nose?
2. Name the passages through which air goes to the lungs.
3. Describe the structure of the lungs.
4. Describe, using a diagram, the processes of inspiration and expiration.
5. Describe what takes place in the air bags of the lungs.
6. How is the size of the chest increased in breathing?

CHAPTER 9

1. What is the work of the blood?
2. Write out in the form of a table the composition of the blood.
3. Describe and give the work of (a) Red Corpuscles,
                                 (b) White Corpuscles.
4. Draw a diagram showing the structure of the heart.
5. Describe briefly the passage of a drop of blood from the Aorta round the body to the Aorta again.
6. Distinguish between arteries, capillaries and veins.
7. Describe the Lymphatic system.

CHAPTER 10

1. Draw a diagram of a tooth showing its structure. Why is it important to keep your teeth clean? How and when do you clean your teeth?
2. Describe the process of digestion in the mouth.
3. Draw a diagram of the stomach, and give an account of the process of digestion in it.
4. What is the work of the liver? What is the composition of bile and what does it do?
5. Describe the process of digestion in the small intestine.
6. Distinguish between " digestion " and " absorption ".
7. What is the structure and work of the large intestine?
8. Explain where and by what means the three main food constituents are digested:—Starches, Proteins, Fats and Oils.

R

CHAPTER 11

1. Give rules for guarding against constipation.
2. Draw a diagram of the kidneys. What is their work?
3. What are the uses of the skin? Draw a diagram showing the structure of the skin.
4. What is the composition of sweat? What is the effect of perspiration?
5. Explain the need of keeping the skin clean.

CHAPTER 12

1. What is the spinal column? What bones are attached to it?
2. Describe the work of the muscles.
3. Where is the nervous system? What is its work?
4. Name the three main sections of the brain and describe their work.
5. Draw a diagram of the eye. Describe its parts.
6. Describe the parts of the ear. How do we keep our balance?
7. In what ways does puberty show itself in boys and girls?

CHAPTER 13

1. What does the word parasite mean? Give three examples of parasites.
2. Write a short account of the connexion between germs and disease.
3. (a) Describe with diagrams three kinds of germs.
   (b) What conditions favour their growth?
4. Give the conditions which hinder the growth of germs. Name some common antiseptics and state how they are used.
5. How do germs enter the body? What takes place when they get inside?
6. Explain carefully the following terms:—Immunity, Inoculation.

CHAPTER 14

1. What is the " Incubation period " of a disease?
   In what diseases is the " Isolation period " most important?
2. What might make you think that a boy or girl had whooping cough. How can it be prevented?
3. How was vaccination against smallpox first discovered?
4. What might make you think that there was the disease called meningitis in your district?

5. What do you know of infantile paralysis (poliomyelitis), and how it can be prevented?
6. What causes tuberculosis? What are the symptoms of TB of the lungs?

CHAPTER 15

1. Give diagrams showing the egg, larva and pupa of the Anopheles mosquito.
2· How can one distinguish between Anopheles and Culex:
    (a) In the egg form?
    (b) in the larva stage?
    (c) In the full-grown insect?
3. Trace the stages by which the cause of malaria was discovered.
4. Give a short account of the life of the malaria parasite in man (give diagrams).
5. Trace the malaria parasite's life in the mosquito.
6. A village, is infested with mosquitoes. If you were given authority how would you attempt to get rid of them?
7. Name some of the medicines which can be taken to prevent and cure malaria.

CHAPTER 16

1. What is the cause of elephantiasis? How is the parasite carried? Give a short life-history of it.
2. Describe some ways of preventing yellow fever from spreading into countries where it is so far unknown.
3. What is relapsing fever? How is it caused?
4. Suppose you are living in a mud house infested with insects. How would you try to get rid of them?
5. Give some account of sleeping sickness. Say what you know of the tsetse fly and give the precautions you would take in travelling through a sleeping sickness country.
6. What do you know of plague? How is it caused? During an epidemic what precautions should be taken by (a) the individual, (b) the town authorities?
7. What habits and dangers of ticks, bedbugs and lice do you know?

CHAPTER 17

1. What is dysentery? How can you protect yourself from this disease?
2. How is cholera spread? How can it be prevented?

3. Describe the course of typhoid fever. What precautions should be taken in a household where there is a typhoid patient?
4. How can sanitation help us to avoid acute bowel diseases?

CHAPTER 18

1. What do you know of (*a*) Roundworms, (*b*) Threadworms, (*c*) ____worms?
2. How ____ the Hookworm spread?
3. What disease is caused by " flukes "? Describe the disease and give an account of the life of a fluke.
4. Give the life-history of the Guinea-worm. How would you treat the disease?
5. Say what you know of Trichina worms.
6. Summarize the ways in which worm diseases can be prevented, stating what diseases can be avoided by each of the methods you mention.
7. Discuss the eating of pork and its dangers, and how to make it safe.

CHAPTER 19

1. What is an ulcer? How would you treat one if you were far from a doctor?
2. What do you know about ringworm? How can it be prevented?
3. How can you recognize the itch (scabies)? How would you treat it?
4. What do you know of leprosy? How can it be stamped out in a country?
5. How would you treat a boil?
6. How can venereal diseases be prevented?
7. Why is " Wash before eating " a good motto?

CHAPTER 20

1. Describe a leptospire. What harm can it do in man?
2. What is the cause of tetanus? How can it be prevented?
3. If you were severely bitten by a dog what would you do? How have some countries been cleared of rabies?
4. Describe fully what you would do if a companion were bitten on the leg by a snake, say on a farm.
5. What precautions would you take when walking in a snake-infested district?

6. A jigger has got into your toe. State clearly what you will do.
7. Why are house-flies dangerous? How can you prevent them breeding?

CHAPTER 21

1. Describe briefly the " water method " of sewage disposal. Give diagrams, including one of a good trap.
2. How are flies kept away from three different latrines that you know?
3. What is the " Dry Pail " System? Describe carefully how such latrines must be kept.
4. Give three common methods for disposal of latrine refuse.
5. What methods are available for the disposal of latrine refuse in a house on a farm? Describe the bore-hole latrine.
6. Give the characteristics of (a) A good dust bin, (b) A good rubbish dump, (c) An incinerator (with a sketch).
7. How can the household refuse of a town be disposed of?

CHAPTER 22

1. What is the best kind of site on which to build a house?
2. Write notes on the construction of a house having regard to (a) the walls, (b) the rooms, (c) the roof, (d) the floors, (e) the windows.
3. In what ways are the surroundings of a house important to health?
4. What is the value of a garden to health?

CHAPTER 23

1. Explain by means of diagrams how land- and sea-breezes are caused.
2. How is climate affected by (a) The Latitude, (b) The Altitude, (c) Rainfall?
3. Write an essay on " Safety First ".
4. Write a short account of the connexion between the climate of a country and the character of its people.
5. Those who know hygiene take more risks. Give reasons for and against this statement.

CHAPTER 24

1. How does the skin lose its heat?
2. What are meant by " good " and " bad " conductors of heat? Give examples.
3. What conditions must clothing satisfy to suit the tropics?

4. Give the characteristics of (*a*) Wool, (*b*) Cotton, as clothing materials.
5. Compare silk and linen. Give the advantages and disadvantages of each as a material for clothes.
6. What is the best kind of head-covering for the tropics? Criticize some of those commonly worn.
7. How does the amount of clothing required vary according to (*a*) Climate, (*b*) Age?

CHAPTER 25

1. What are the effects of moderate exercise?
2. Give the bad effects of (*a*) Over-exercise, (*b*) Lack of exercise.
3. Why should all boys and girls take some part in sport? Give some rules concerning sport and exercise.
4. Why is rest necessary? Give some rules concerning sleep.
5. Explain carefully the importance to health of the formation of regular habits. Illustrate your answer by reference to Sleep, Meals, Bowel action and Care of Teeth.
6. Why should care be taken of the hair and finger-nails?
7. What signs would lead us to suspect a boy's eyesight is defective?
8. A boy's eyes are sore and red and there is a white discharge. What will you do and what avoid?
9. How can the spread of eye disease be prevented?
10. Why should a discharge from the ears be considered a serious thing?

CHAPTER 26

1. Give rules for stopping bleeding.
2. How would you try to stop a boy's nose bleeding?
3. A boy cuts his foot while digging in a garden. Explain carefully what you would do.
4. What are the signs of fracture?
5. What are splints used for? How could you make one in an emergency?
6. A boy falls off a bicycle and breaks his shin-bone. What aid could you render? Where would you do it?
7. Describe the treatment for (*a*) A sprain, (*b*) A burn or scald.
8. How would you help a boy whose clothes had caught fire?
9. A boy is pulled out of the water apparently drowned. How would you act?
10. How would you distinguish between a fainting fit and a case of heatstroke?
11. What are the general rules for treatment in case of poisoning?

CHAPTER 27

1. Why does the government concern itself about our health? Is it not the duty of our parents?
2. Name some of the activities of the Health Service which are going on near your own home.
3. What does a Health Inspector have to do?
4. Why are Vital Statistics important?
5. What does " Notification " mean? Name some diseases which you think ought to be notified.
6. What kind of a job in the Health Service would you like to do? Explain why.

INDEX

Number of page with fullest description of the item is in heavy type

245